Inflation and the Economic Well-being of the Elderly

Inflation and the Economic Well-being of the Elderly

Robert L. Clark
George L. Maddox
Ronald A. Schrimper
Daniel A. Sumner

The Johns Hopkins University Press
Baltimore and London

The Johns Hopkins University Press, Baltimore, Maryland 21218
The Johns Hopkins Press Ltd., London

The paper in this book is acid-free and meets the guidelines
for permanence and durability of the Committee on
Production Guidelines for Book Longevity of the
Council on Library Resources.

Library of Congress Cataloging in Publication Data
Main entry under title:

Inflation and the economic well-being of the elderly.

  Bibliography: pp. 131–36
  Includes index.
  1. Aged — United States — Economic conditions.
2. Cost and standard of living — United States. 3. Old
age assistance — United States. 4. Income — United States
— Effect of inflation on. I. Clark, Robert Louis,
1949–
HQ1064.U5I54   1984   305.2'6'0973   84–7863
ISBN 0–8018–3218–7   (alk. paper)

Contents

LIST OF FIGURES

LIST OF TABLES

Acknowledgments

We acknowledge the important contributions of several people who assisted in the preparation of this book. James Leiby, Deborah McConnell, Laurence M. Wallman, and Stephan Gohmann provided excellent research assistance for the project. Wallman made a distinctive contribution to the analysis of health expenditures presented in Chapter 8. Mary Jane Gorman contributed the analysis of the Panel Study of Income Dynamics in Chapter 4. Daphne O'Neal and Deborah Coley typed and edited several drafts of the manuscript. Ann Phillips also assisted with the final editing and Peggy Hoover served as copy editor for Johns Hopkins University Press. The National Institute on Aging supported the research reported here (Grant No. 1 R01 AG 02345-01). Additional support for our analysis was provided by the North Carolina Agricultural Research Service.

Introduction

The causes and effects of high rates of inflation significantly influenced events during the late 1970s and set the stage for anti-inflationary policies during the 1980s. Although the rate of inflation fell during the early 1980s, the effect of inflation on real income and the distribution of income remains an important issue. This book examines the well-being of older Americans during the 1970s and seeks to determine how inflation affected that well-being. We have analyzed a series of surveys to determine shifts in real income and consumption and have studied the sources of income of the elderly to identify general responses to rising prices. This methodology could be applied to any demographic group; the elderly were chosen because of widespread concern that they are vulnerable to loss of real income due to inflation. In addition, because older persons receive a substantial portion of their income from government transfers, the effect of inflation on their real income has important public policy implications.

It has long been believed that the elderly are more adversely affected by inflation than are other demographic groups. For example, at the beginning of the 1970s, Arthur Okun (1970, p. 14) concluded that the "retired aged are the only major specific demographic group of Americans that I can confidently identify as income losers" in response to inflation. Illustrating the continuing prevalence of this view is the final report of the 1981 White House Conference on Aging, which stated that "the elderly are particularly vulnerable to loss from inflation" and that "reduced inflation is especially beneficial to retired persons because it allows them to be better able to take care of themselves and affords the economy more output to share with needy nonworkers" (pp. 27, 30).

In this book we carefully examine and then reject the hypothesis that the elderly are more vulnerable to inflation. The flaw in the argument that they are vulnerable to inflation is the assumption that older persons live on fixed incomes — which they do not. In the recent past the major income sources of the elderly have been earnings, social security payments, pensions, other federal transfer programs, and returns on accumulated assets. The wages and interest rates that the elderly earn rise with expected inflation just as they do for the rest of the population. Explicit indexation, ad hoc adjustments, and in-kind benefit payments have maintained the real value of federally administered transfers to the elderly. Employer pension benefits also tend to rise with inflation, although these do not seem to have kept pace with price increases. Finally, informal transfers from family and consumption from accumulated durable assets are difficult to measure, but they are a significant factor in the well-being of the elderly. Since most sources of income for the elderly are not fixed but increase along with price increases, the real issues are the change in income relative to changes in the prices of goods the elderly purchase and relative to incomes of other groups, and the diversity in consumption patterns and income among older persons.

Chapters 1–3 outline the conceptual issues involved in understanding and measuring changes in well-being. In Chapter 1, family well-being is assumed to be determined by available resources and current market prices. The effect of inflation on well-being depends on changes in the relative prices of goods consumed as compared with changes in prices of family resources and wages of family members. In Chapter 2 we apply this model to the elderly in a discussion of their sources of income and the goods they consume. Chapter 3 examines and compares alternative measures of inflation. The consumer price index, the personal consumption expenditure price index, and three types of budgets for retired couples are described. Trends in each of these indicators are presented to illustrate the rising prices of the 1970s. We also review studies that constructed separate price indexes for older persons. As a result of this analysis, we chose the consumer price index as the primary measure of inflation for this study.

The changing nominal and real income of the elderly is reported in Chapters 4–6. Chapter 4 derives age-income relationships for individuals in two longitudinal surveys, which follow the same individuals over time and show how they respond to aging and the changing economic environment. In contrast to this life-cycle income pattern of individuals, the income of specific age groups is examined. The distinction between examining the changing income of a cohort of individuals as they age and the income of a specific age group as it changes over time is very important in understanding the trend in the well-being of older persons. Throughout the following chapters, both these concepts are employed to indicate changes in the real income of the elderly.

The growth and development of government income maintenance programs are outlined in Chapter 5. Expansion of these programs during the 1960s and 1970s has resulted in an increasing proportion of the elderly's income being derived from public sources. The responsiveness of earnings, social security, and pensions to price changes is examined in Chapter 6. These are the three most important sources of income to the elderly, so an understanding of how they respond to inflation is important.

Expenditure patterns of older persons are the focus of Chapters 7–8. In Chapter 7 we employ the 1972–73 Consumer Expenditure Survey to derive the proportion of family income devoted to specific commodity groups and note significant differences across age groups. We use the more limited consumption data of the Retirement History Study to supplement these findings. Chapter 7 also indicates the important distinction between the changing well-being of an age group composed of different individuals over time and changes in the well-being of a cohort whose composition changes only with mortality. Because of the importance of medical care to the elderly, Chapter 8 focuses solely on health expenditures, using the Retirement History Study.

The final chapter reviews the findings of the Retirement History Study and assesses the potential inflation effects on the well-being of the elderly. Future inflation effects will be governed by the economic responses and institutional constraints examined in this study. We analyze possible future effects on well-being by considering the changing political and economic environment.

This book is concerned with the well-being of older persons during the 1970s. Data over a longer period provide a long-run perspective on the trend in the well-being of the elderly. Changes in income from government programs and work rates of older persons during the 1970s are really continuations of trends. Evidence from the early 1980s shows whether the improving well-being of the 1970s is continuing into the 1980s. Thus, this book's examination of a recent inflationary period shows how the well-being of older persons has been influenced by rising prices. This experience is carefully analyzed to determine how income and expenditures responded to price increases, and these responses are assessed to determine how price increases in the future will affect the elderly in a changed political and economic environment.

Currently there is political debate over whether to reduce the inflation protection provided to older persons through federal programs. Reducing or eliminating the automatic increase of social security benefits and cutbacks in transfer programs could alter the response of income of the elderly to price increases. The important role that governmental policy played in raising the real income for most older adults in the 1970s implies that findings in this book may be altered if governmental policies change.

Inflation and the Economic Well-being of the Elderly

1 The Concept of Well-being and Its Relationship to Inflation

The concept of individual well-being has been the focus of research in many disciplines. In this book we employ standard economic theory that relates well-being to potential consumption of goods and services. Potential consumption is limited by real income and commodity prices, which may be affected by inflation. We begin our study by providing a framework for analyzing the effect of inflation on the well-being of the elderly in later chapters.

A MEASURE OF WELL-BEING

In order to examine the effect of inflation on the well-being of a group of people, one must have some measure of well-being. As a practical basis for comparison, we have adopted the principles of a subjective utility or satisfaction index as a general measure of well-being. Individuals and families are assumed to allocate their productive resources to earn income and to allocate their income and time among goods and services in order to make themselves as well-off as possible. Much of economics is derived from considering preferences in relation to prices and endowments to explain behavior. Textbook treatments of utility theory are contained in Miller (1982), Mansfield (1979), Layard and Walters (1978), and Henderson and Quandt (1980). The concept of economic well-being is discussed and applied in Moon (1977) and Moon and Smolensky (1977).

The well-being of an individual depends on the levels of consumption of goods and services. Our concept of goods and services is very broad and includes such standard items as housing, health care, or food but also time spent with children or quality of intracity transportation. Each of the goods and services available contributes to the well-being of the consumer. However, goods and services may substitute for one another; for example, reducing the consumption of housing by some degree while increasing the consumption of medical services may leave a consumer equally well-off. More of both goods is preferred to less, but more of one may compensate for less of the other. In terms of producing well-being, various goods and services that people consume are substitutable; they may be combined in different proportions to yield the same level of satisfaction.

1

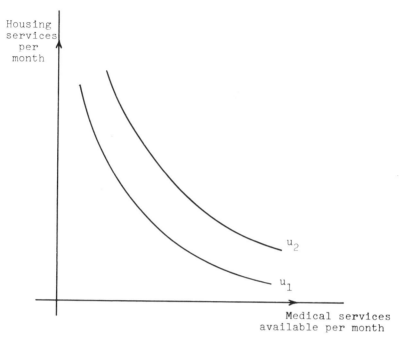

FIGURE 1.1. The Index of Well-being, Illustrated

As a further proposition, the more one consumes of a given commodity, the less of some other desirable commodity is required to substitute per unit while leaving well-being constant. For example, at low levels of housing service it would take a larger increase in medical services to compensate for further reduction in the quantity of housing than it would at higher levels of housing service consumption.

The idea of the index of well-being (U) is illustrated in Figure 1.1. Quantities of two goods, say, housing and medical services, are shown on the vertical and horizontal axes. Increasing both goods entails moving in a northeastern direction. Two levels of well-being are shown in the figure. The index U_2 represents more consumption and so a higher level of well-being than U_1; that is, the consumer prefers U_2 to U_1. Each U index slopes down to the right and is convex. Movement along the curve U_2 indicates alternative combinations of the two goods that provide the same level of well-being.

In the basic economic model of consumer behavior, only consumption of goods affects a person's well-being. There is no allowance for changing the preferences themselves. Although this may seem to be a narrow view of human behavior, a broad array of goods and services may be included.

Because income itself is not an item of consumption, it influences well-being only by affecting levels of consumption of the various desirable goods

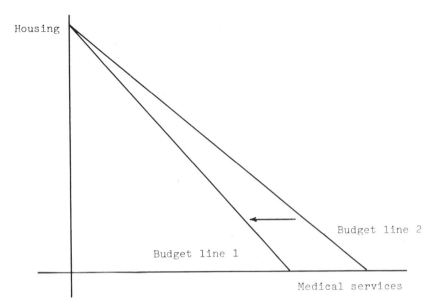

FIGURE 1.2. The Consumer Budget, Illustrated

and services. Of course, consumption and hence the level of well-being is limited by income. A consumer's budget represents an equation in which the sum of all income earned from various sources and other claims to resources must be balanced against all the expenditures for consumption of goods and services. The external economic environment of the individual affects well-being by affecting the consumer's budget. Given some potential amount of work time, a set of skills and marketable abilities, and an endowment of other assets and resources, the wage rate, rates of return on investments, and other prices determine the consumer's potential income. Prices of various goods and services determine the level of consumption and therefore well-being that the individual may attain.

The consumer's best choice of goods and services is the one that makes well-being as great as possible while not making total expenditures greater than total income. The objective and external economic environment is represented by the consumer's wage and rates of return that determine total income and by the prices of the goods and services that determine the budget constraint. Changes in the economy affect well-being by changing the income the consumer has to spend or by changing the prices of the goods and services among which the consumer's income is allocated.

An individual's budget is illustrated in Figure 1.2. Consumption goods are shown on the vertical and horizontal axes. The Budget Line 2 shows the potential consumption at an initial set of prices and income. A proportionate

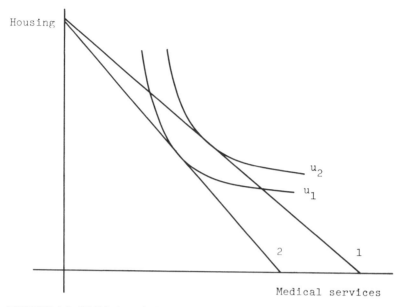

FIGURE 1.3. Well-being Limited by the Consumer's Budget

increase in both prices or a fall in the income would shift the budget line toward the origin in a parallel fashion. In the figure, Budget Line 1 shows potential consumption of each good after a rise in the price of medical services, while the price of housing and the consumer's income were held fixed. This illustrates that less of either good may be purchased except at the point where all income was being spent on housing. Increasing the price of some good reduces well-being because it reduces potential consumption of all goods.

Figure 1.3 combines the representation of consumer preferences and well-being of Figure 1.1 with the representation of the consumer budget of Figure 1.2. The change in consumption in response to an increase in the price of medical services is derived from two conceptually separable forces. First, the price of medical services has risen relative to the price of housing, causing a substitution of housing for medical services. Second, the price of medical services has risen relative to consumer income, reducing real purchasing power. This further reduces consumption of most goods.

The above model of a consumer allocating income to achieve the highest possible level of well-being given available levels of wealth, income, and time provides a theoretical framework to enhance the interpretation of the data presented in subsequent chapters. The average price level determines real income, and relative prices indicate the cost of one good in terms of other goods. Increases in the average price level will lower real income (resulting in an inward shift of the budget constraint) unless nominal income rises by an equal or greater amount.

INFLATION

Most transactions in the U.S. economy use dollars to measure the goods and services being traded. Absolute or money prices are the rates of exchange between dollars and particular goods and services. The general price level or the level of the price index is an average level of the money prices in an economy, but this average price level must be compared with something to be meaningful. Typically, the general price level is compared to past levels or to prices in other nations or regions.

Inflation is the sustained increase in the general level of prices measured against some monetary unit. It might be thought of as a shrinking of the measuring rod we use to measure incomes and expenditures. To say that the prices of goods and services in general have risen is to say that the value of a unit of money has fallen.

An inflation rate is measured as the rate of change of some index of prices per unit of time. If an average of the prices of some group of goods and services rises from 100 to 110 in a year, the inflation rate for that year is 10 percent. An increase in inflation is an increase in the *rate* at which prices are rising, not an increase in the prices themselves. Inflation may be falling while prices are rising. Recently, the press has begun referring to this phenomenon as disinflation.

Relative prices are the rates at which goods and services may be traded for each other; thus they are the ratios of money prices. For example, if a bus ride across town costs 50¢ whereas a taxi ride costs $3, the relative price is six bus rides for one taxi ride. Pure inflation that raised the bus ticket to $1 and the taxi ride to $6 has no effect on these relative prices. One problem with inflation is that it is often difficult to distinguish relative price changes from inflation.

Variations in the inflation rate from year to year mean that any adjustments to inflation must also vary from year to year. In order to make reasonable decisions in the allocation of their scarce resources, people must gather information about the relative prices in the economy. When the price of bus rides changes *relative* to the price of taxi rides, people are likely to rearrange their consumption. If some nominal price rises, a consumer may not know whether prices are rising generally or if the relative price of this good alone has risen.

Information about price changes is valuable and not free, and so consumers and producers will use resources to find out how prices have changed. For example, a worker who received a wage increase may not know if the wages of workers in other firms or occupations have risen. He may then not know without searching in the labor market whether a change of employers would be in his interest. Especially with variable rates of inflation, the costs of gathering price information and the cost of mistakes in allocation may be sizable.

INFLATION AND WELL-BEING

If all prices rose together in exact proportion, and if we all knew that this was happening, inflation would have little effect because we would design our institutions and transactions so that the influence of nominal price changes would be nullified. In Figure 1.3, if all prices and income were to increase in proportion, there would be no change in the budget lines and the same well-being index would be attained. But relative prices do change, and uncertainty with respect to price changes does exist. The model illustrated above does not consider the cost of gathering information about price changes. A more complete model would incorporate information as one of the goods that people purchase. Consider the effects of price changes that were not correctly measured by a consumer. The level of well-being would be below its maximum potential level, and consumption patterns would fail to adjust fully to the new relative prices because the price changes would not be fully detected.

When people have the opportunity to substitute goods that have become cheaper for goods that have become more expensive, they often can mitigate negative effects of price changes. In fact, if nominal prices and incomes change in a way that leaves the original consumption bundle available, the consumer could always be better off after the price change. However, in a world in which information about price changes is not free and there are costs associated with changing consumption proportions, price changes may leave a consumer worse off, at least in the short run before substitution takes place.

In any economy, relative prices of goods and services are constantly changing. Wages and other determinants of consumer incomes also change. In response, people change the quantities of goods and services bought and sold, and they change hours of work, occupations, and other determinants of income. When inflation is added to the normal movements in relative prices, it means that while nominal prices move up and down relative to one another, the average tendency is for prices to rise. This added movement will tend to make mistakes occur more frequently and this constitutes a real cost of inflation in the economy (Dornbusch and Fischer, 1981; Gordon, 1981).

THE USE OF PRICE INDEXES
TO MEASURE CHANGES IN WELL-BEING

Changes in the level of prices in general are usually measured using some form of weighted average. In computing the average price level, the price of each commodity is weighted by the budget share of that commodity in consumers' market baskets. These expenditure shares are not easy to measure in practice, but they have a clear conceptual basis at this level of generality. (See Chapter 2 for a discussion of a budget share for the elderly in empirical application. See Chapter 3 for important details about particular price indexes.)

If we take the budget shares as fixed, the change in the average price level implied by changes in specific commodity prices may be calculated as the sum of the individual percentage price changes each weighted by its budget share. Usually the base period average price level is defined as 100.0, so the change in the average price level is equivalent to a percentage change. If, for example, we wish to calculate the change in the price index between 1980 and 1981, each of the individual price changes refers to the price of goods in 1981 minus the price of the goods in 1980 in percentage terms. If used only to indicate how a particular weighted average of prices has changed, this technique poses no problems. Often, however, the inflation rate calculated in this way relative to changes in consumer incomes is used to approximate changes in consumer well-being. Thus, the ratio of changes in income to changes in the price index is used to determine the change in consumer well-being. If this ratio is less than 1.0, consumer prices have risen by more than consumer income, and so fewer goods and services can be bought.

There are two basic conceptual problems with using the average change in consumer prices relative to the change in income to measure the changes in well-being. First, all consumers do not buy the same bundle of goods and services, so the shares of income spent on each good or service are different. This means that the average change relevant to one person is not relevant to others who have different expenditure shares. For example, if Smith has a high share of housing relative to Jones and the price of housing increased more than other prices, the weighted average price change relevant to Smith has gone up by more than that relevant to Jones. Usually inflation is measured using some average shares in the initial time period for the calculations. People who consume more than an average amount of the goods for which prices have risen must actually face a higher relevant inflation rate than the measured one. This may be especially important for the elderly, whose average expenditure pattern differs from that of other age groups. (See Chapter 7 for a discussion of differences in budget shares by age and Chapter 3 for a review of age-specific price indexes.)

The second problem inherent in using the weighted average change in prices in calculating changes in well-being is that the budget shares will not be constant when prices change. A consumer's allocation of income among goods and services tends to change over time because of several forces, for example aging or changing family structure. Also, changes in budget shares are inherent in relative price changes themselves. Thus, when there is an inflation and the prices rise differentially, the shares relevant at the beginning of the period will no longer be relevant at the end of the period. As in the models above, consumers tend to substitute away from goods whose prices have risen the most. Because consumers tend to substitute among goods in response to relative price changes, the loss in consumer well-being may be overstated by the normal measures of inflation.

2 Income and Expenditures of the Elderly

Now we can build on the model outlined in Chapter 1 by applying the concepts developed there to the specific case of the elderly in the current U.S. economic environment. This chapter will provide a research strategy to project the impact of inflation on both income and expenditures using the concept of the consumer budget as the basic model.

APPLYING A MODEL OF WELL-BEING TO THE EFFECTS OF INFLATION ON THE ELDERLY

Any household has both income and expenditures. With various adjustments for saving and borrowing to smooth consumption over time, one can establish a balance between income from endowments of resources (like work-time and skills) and expenditures on consumption items (like housing or medical services). In such a budget relationship, income may be thought of as the sum of the price multiplied by the quantity of each income source that is sold during the period. This may include the wage rate multiplied by hours of work to yield earnings, but also owned housing units rented multipled by rent per period to yield rental income. For owner-occupied housing (or other major durable goods) for which no external transaction takes place, it is useful to think of households renting the living space to themselves, yielding both income and expenditures. Income in the form of gifts or other transfers should be included as part of family income, with the unit value of the transfer included as one of the prices faced by the household.

Total expenditures may also be thought of as the sum of the price multiplied by the quantity of each good. These include not only straightforward consumption items like food or rent but also implicit consumption of owner-occupied housing and consumption of transfers of goods and services to the household. These transfer items given and received are especially important for the elderly and are discussed more fully below and in Chapter 5.

Our measure of the well-being of the elderly depends directly on the quantity of the various items consumed. Price changes affect well-being by affecting these quantities of goods and services consumed. On the income side of the budget, price changes of consumption items affect how far the income will go in providing total well-being to the household and which items are relatively most expensive.

If all prices of income sources and consumption goods and services increased by the same proportion between two periods, the budget equation would still be balanced, with no change in any of the quantities of sources of income or quantities of goods consumed. Ignoring costs of information and uncertainty, we note that changes in well-being are associated with changes in the goods consumed, so if there are no changes in the consumption of goods, pure inflation has no effect on well-being. Inflation has an effect on consumption if it changes relative prices. For example, if the prices of goods rise by more than the prices of income sources, the budget will be unbalanced unless lower quantities are consumed. Over any particular period, relative prices will change, benefiting some people and hurting others.

The rate of inflation does not enter directly into a budget equation. In fact, with all prices rising at the same rate in a long-run equilibrium, with complete and accurate anticipations of the inflation rate and full institutional adjustment, there would be little or no impact even if the rate of inflation were high. In understanding the overall effects of inflation, there are several major problems: (a) the inflation rate is not fully anticipated, (b) the rate of price increases varies greatly, (c) there is uncertainty about actual rates and confusion between relative price changes and overall inflation, and (d), an important corollary to the above, institutions do not adjust quickly or without cost to an environment of high and variable inflation rates. If high rates of inflation persist, then perceptions, expectations, and institutions would more fully reflect potential inflation, and its effect would be different. This important distinction between anticipated inflation and actual inflation should be kept in mind in any discussion of the effect of inflation. In addition, it raises problems in generalizing from past inflations to the potential effects of actual future inflations. These problems are addressed directly in Chapter 9.

INCOME OF THE ELDERLY

The major sources of income in households of the elderly in the United States are labor market earnings, employer pensions, social security, interest and dividends and other asset income, government cash transfers, private cash transfers, in-kind private transfers, in-kind government transfers, and the use of consumer durables. The above list could be expanded, and for some purposes this would be useful. Some of these income sources are effectively fixed in the current period, being based on past choices and circumstances, whereas others are responsive to current decisions. The choice variables may be adjusted to changes in the economic environment facing the family (such as changes in actual or anticipated rate of inflation); the fixed sources respond to changes in the economic environment only through institutional or other channels outside the family's direct control. This distinction is vital for understanding the income, well-being, and economic behavior of the elderly in inflationary periods.

The elderly are distinguished from others by different shares of income that come from each of the sources, and subpopulations of the elderly have different shares of their total income coming from each of these sources. For example, almost all persons over the age of 65 receive some social security payments, but the share of social security income varies widely among the elderly; for some it is the major income source, for others it is only a minor supplement. Given the recent indexing of social security payments, this is important. Another income source almost universal among the elderly is medicare benefits, which form a part of the in-kind government transfers. How important medicare is to the elderly depends on the amount of total income and on the health of the elderly family. Since this transfer is an in-kind benefit, it is also effectively protected from inflation. Note that the relative price of the commodity is affected by the form of the transfer, which is true for all in-kind transfers.

Income sources in the form of specified quantities of consumed goods and services are particularly difficult to evaluate. Consider medical services as an example. A household eligible for medicare has received a low- (perhaps zero-) priced insurance plan. Part of the household resources is the value of this insurance. But even if a market value of the insurance could be established, there is the additional problem that some households would not have purchased such private insurance at that price. Thus, their income would be overestimated by valuing medicare at its market value. (For an assessment of the value of in-kind benefits, see Chapter 5, Moon [1977], Moon and Smolensky [1977], Paglin [1980], and Smeeding [1982].)

Many income sources do not depend directly on the current choices of the elderly (e.g., in response to inflation), but work behavior is usually under the control of the individual. The choice to retire or to change hours of work or employment commitment will be affected by the effect of inflation on other income and on the prices of goods. On the average, wage rates would be expected to grow with inflation, but this is not true for all groups. Also, as we will see below, the value of pension benefits and the decision to accept pensions may be affected in a major way by current and anticipated rates of inflation. When the prices of assets and durables change, this change in wealth affects potential consumption and well-being in each period even if the asset is not sold and the capital gain is not realized. Take housing services as an example, and consider a family that owns its home. Part of the total income of this family is the service flow in each period from the house. The family housing expenditure includes use of this house (rather than renting or selling it). Now consider unanticipated increases in the price of houses over time. This capital gain increases the value of durable assets, and this increases "total" income. On the expenditure side, it also increases the value of the service flow of housing received.

These examples illustrate that inflation may affect the elderly differently from other families and that this effect will not be homogeneous among different segments of the elderly population. The amounts and shares of income received from each source, and the decisions about work and other investments, determine these differential impacts. We have not fully discussed how inflation might affect each of the income sources, and we have not indicated definitely the expected responses. Chapters 4 and 5 examine the pattern of income changes, and Chapter 6 gives special attention to how earnings, pension benefits, and social security benefits respond to changes in consumer prices. The discussion here is meant to be merely illustrative and to indicate how the data in subsequent chapters should be assessed.

EXPENDITURES OF THE ELDERLY

Consumption patterns of the elderly are different from those of the rest of the population. Consumption may be purchased goods and services, private in-kind transfers, government in-kind transfers, service flows from consumer durables, net savings, and taxes and government services. Purchased goods and services pose no new conceptual problems, although careful measurements of prices and quantities of these items is often difficult. Within this category the elderly tend to spend more for some items than for others, relative to younger families with physical and wealth differences.

In-kind transfers from private or governmental sources, discussed above as income sources, also appear as separate expenditure categories, because recipients cannot move the grant freely into other forms of consumption. If the in-kind transfer is at a level lower than the household would have consumed in absence of the transfer, the household will make additional expenditures and the total budget for that category is accurately reflected by the sum of the in-kind and supplemental expenditures. The amount of transfers is often larger than the household would have purchased, and this is a major rationale for in-kind transfers. In this case, the additional constraint on the household budget allocation must be examined carefully.

Given stocks of assets at the beginning of a period and transfers during the period, the basic decisions the consumer makes are a consumption-savings decision (that is, how much to add or subtract from net wealth) and a portfolio decision (that is, allocating savings or dissavings between productive assets and consumer durables). The consumer also decides how to allocate all current consumption among the potential goods and services. Savings decisions are life-cycle choices that depend crucially on expected length of life. They also depend on the real expected rate of return on investments after effects of anticipated inflation are subtracted out. Allocation of consumption depends on the total income to be allocated, the whole set of prices, and the other constraints that may be placed on the household. An example of these other constraints might be the amount of in-kind income.

The savings decision of a household depends on the expected inflation-adjusted interest rate for each period in the future, and other factors unique to that household. Inflation anticipation affects savings by potentially affecting the real rate of interest and perhaps the other variables. Inflation may alter the current consumption mix by affecting relative prices, real current income, or other constraints that apply to the household.

The issue of taxes is usually dealt with either by using net after-tax income or by letting taxes be a separate expenditure category. If income tax payments are thought of as a payment for services from the government, then gross income should be the measure of income, and tax payments should be included as one of the expenditure categories. The problem is that no separation of price from quantity is possible. No calculation of the increases in the price of government services is possible.

In developing the empirical evidence about expenditure patterns (see Chapters 7 and 8), several practical issues are important. Because information on price and quantities of some goods is not available, researchers must either leave some categories out of the analysis or treat those categories as a residual that is not analyzed. This incompleteness causes unavoidable problems. The aggregation of goods into manageable categories is also often arbitrary and is determined largely by data availability. Principles of aggregation are, briefly, that goods should be closely related in the sense that they substitute closely for one another or that they are used in fixed proportions. Also, relative price movements within an aggregate should be at a minimum. For example, if the price of physicians goes up and the price of drugs goes down, consumer response will be masked if an aggregate medical services category is used. In this case, if one group of consumers uses more physician services and fewer drugs, the differential impact between groups will be hidden.

In developing the household budget, the amount of time away from work which people have to devote to consumption is not included, but it may be an important source of well-being and is not ignored in our comparisons of the elderly with younger people. Further, some expenditures are a function of how income itself is generated; for example, commuting costs or the cost of work uniforms depend on holding a job. In comparing incomes or welfare across groups, it is appropriate to account for such costs. For the self-employed, business costs must be subtracted from gross receipts before income is used in consumption analysis; the same applies to those with income from employment or assets. These issues are especially important in comparing the elderly with other groups and are discussed further in Chapter 9.

The two sides of the family budget constraint provide the structure for this book. Trends in income and specific income sources during the 1970s (examined in Chapters 4–6) and expenditure changes over the same period (see Chapters 7 and 8) are factors to consider in determining the influence of inflation on well-being. The model developed in these first two chapters can help explain gains in well-being during the 1970s and serve as a guide for understanding potential inflation effects in the 1980s.

3 Measuring Inflation: Price Indexes and Budgets

In order to determine changes in real income, the trend in nominal income must be adjusted for increases in the price level. This deflated or real income indicates whether purchasing power has been affected (see Chapter 1). In this chapter we describe price indexes that can be used to measure inflation and thus to assess changes in the real income of the elderly. One of these indexes, the consumer price index, is adopted as the measure of inflation used throughout subsequent chapters to determine trends in real income. In addition, we assess the usefulness of three retired-couple budgets as indicators of the economic well-being of the elderly.

THE CONSUMER PRICE INDEX

The consumer price index (CPI) is probably the most widely used measure of inflation. Many labor contracts and the social security program use the CPI to escalate income payments to maintain a constant standard of living. The consumer price index measures the change in the value of a fixed market basket of goods and services over time. This allows comparisons of consumption from one period to another, since the quantity purchased in the base period for the market basket remains unchanged. A problem with this index is that because people do not continue to buy the same quantities after changes in relative prices (see Chapter 1), this index overestimates the number of dollars required to remain at the same satisfaction level as the base period by not considering the effects of substitution. This complicates use of the CPI as a cost-of-living index. Most studies indicate, however, that the magnitude of this bias is fairly small (Braithwait, 1980; Triplett, 1981; and Cagan and Moore, 1981). Another problem is that the CPI also excludes taxes and in-kind consumption and may not completely adjust for quality changes in products. Despite these shortcomings, however, the CPI is still used for cost-of-living adjustments because the purpose of these adjustments is to permit people to purchase the quantities of goods they purchased in a base period, thereby leaving them at least as well-off as they were.

Current CPI measurements are based on consumption patterns reflected in the 1972–73 Consumer Expenditure Survey conducted by the U.S. Bureau of Labor Statistics. The market basket has been revised every ten to twelve years

15

TABLE 3.1. Consumer Price Index and Some of Its Major Components for Urban Wage Earners and Clerical Workers, 1967–82

Year	Total	Food and Beverages	Housing	Medical Care
1967	100.0	100.0	100.0	100.0
1968	104.2	103.6	104.0	106.1
1969	109.8	108.8	110.4	113.4
1970	116.3	114.7	118.2	120.6
1971	121.3	118.3	123.4	128.4
1972	125.3	123.2	128.1	132.5
1973	133.1	139.5	133.7	137.7
1974	147.7	158.7	148.8	150.5
1975	161.2	172.1	164.5	168.6
1976	170.5	177.4	174.6	184.7
1977	181.5	188.0	186.5	202.4
1978	195.3	206.2	202.6	219.4
1979	217.7	228.7	227.5	240.1
1980	247.0	248.7	263.2	267.2
1981	272.3	267.8	293.2	295.1
1982	288.6	278.5	314.7	326.9

Source: U.S. Bureau of Labor Statistics, *Monthly Labor Review,* March 1983, table 18.

to adjust for changes in expenditure patterns caused by relative price changes among products, the introduction of new products, the disappearance of old products, shifts in tastes, and other socioeconomic variables. Each month prices are collected in 85 urban areas from about 24,000 establishments for the items included in the 1972–73 market basket. The 1972–73 market basket for urban wage earners and clerical workers contains the following weights by component: food, 20.4 percent; housing, 39.8 percent; apparel, 7.0 percent; transportation, 19.9 percent; medical care, 4.2 percent; entertainment, 3.4 percent; personal care, 1.8 percent. The weights for all urban consumers are: food, 18.8 percent; housing, 42.9 percent; apparel, 7.0 percent; transportation, 17.7 percent; medical care, 4.6 percent; entertainment, 4.5 percent; personal care, 1.7 percent (Cagan and Moore, 1981).

Starting in 1978 the Bureau of Labor Statistics began publishing two consumer price indexes based on the alternative sets of weights. Since the differences in weights are relatively small, both indexes have indicated approximately the same rate of inflation since that period.

The CPI indexes are published monthly for the United States and the five metropolitan areas by the Bureau of Labor Statistics. Other values published bimonthly are regional and city-size indexes and twenty-three other large metropolitan area indexes. The latter indexes reflect changes over time in the base period's consumption in each geographical area. They do not indicate differences in price levels or costs of living among areas. The trend in the CPI from 1967 to 1982, along with the trend in the major components, is presented in Table 3.1. The annual percentage increases are indicated in Table 3.2.

TABLE 3.2. Percentage Changes in Consumer Price Index by Component, 1968–82

	1968	1969	1970	1971	1972	1973	1974	
All items	4.2	5.4	5.9	4.3	3.3	6.2	11.0	
Food and beverages	3.6	5.0	5.4	3.1	4.1	13.2	13.8	
Housing	4.0	6.2	7.1	4.4	3.8	4.4	11.3	
Apparel and upkeep	5.4	5.8	4.1	3.2	2.1	3.7	7.4	
Transportation	3.2	3.9	5.1	5.2	1.1	3.3	11.2	
Medical care	6.1	6.9	6.3	6.5	3.2	3.9	9.3	
Entertainment	5.7	5.0	5.1	5.3	2.9	2.8	7.5	
Other goods and services	5.2	4.9	5.8	4.8	4.2	3.9	7.2	

	1975	1976	1977	1978	1979	1980	1981	1982
All items	9.1	5.8	6.5	7.6	11.5	13.5	10.2	6.0
Food and beverages	8.4	3.1	6.0	9.7	10.9	8.7	7.7	4.0
Housing	10.6	6.1	6.8	8.6	12.3	15.7	11.4	7.3
Apparel and upkeep	4.5	3.7	4.5	3.4	4.3	6.6	5.2	2.3
Transportation	9.4	9.9	7.1	4.9	14.5	17.7	12.3	4.2
Medical care	12.0	9.5	9.6	8.4	9.4	11.3	10.4	10.8
Entertainment	8.9	5.0	4.9	5.1	6.5	8.5	7.5	6.1
Other goods and services	8.4	5.7	5.8	6.4	7.2	8.8	9.2	10.2

Source: Bureau of Labor Statistics, *Monthly Labor Review,* March 1983, table 18.

PERSONAL CONSUMPTION EXPENDITURE
IMPLICIT PRICE DEFLATOR

The personal consumption expenditure implicit price deflator (PCE) compares a current market basket of commodities and services at current prices to the value of an identical set of goods at the base-year prices. The PCE reflects changes in consumption patterns in response to relative price changes. Since the index reflects changing market baskets of goods and services, meaningful comparisons can be made only between current prices and prices in the base period. Such an index can be used to measure the change in price between any two given points in time, but successive values of the index do not accurately reflect changes in annual inflation rates over a period of time. A more complete discussion of this issue is presented in Triplett (1981).

An index like the PCE tends to change at a slower rate than a base-year weighted price index like the CPI, because the changes in the weights of the PCE reflect substitutions that consumers make among goods and services in response to relative price changes. Consequently, the PCE tends to understate inflation. If consumers have shifted toward the use of goods that have fallen in relative price, then the PCE will understate the rise in prices consumers experience.

The PCE is derived from data collected on personal consumption expenditures as part of the national income and product accounts developed by the U.S. Department of Commerce. The index is based on the value of new and used goods and services purchased by all urban and rural individuals, operating expenses of nonprofit institutions, and the value of food, rent, clothing, and financial services received as in-kind benefits by individuals. Expenditure data for the various components are deflated by an appropriate price index, which in many cases is a component of the CPI. The deflated components are then added together to get the value in constant dollars for the base period (Schwenk, 1981).

The aggregate monthly expenditure estimates are divided into durable and nondurable goods categories. The value of services is estimated from receipts by service industries, reports of financial institutions, employment and earnings in service-related industries, and consumer stocks of durable goods and resident housing. Total personal expenditures for food, housing, medical care, transportation, clothing, and all other items are shown in Table 3.3. These data, which are collected monthly, are the basis for the PCE deflator. The PCE is published monthly and is revised regularly as estimates of expenditures are adjusted. The values of this index from 1967 to 1982 are indicated in Table 3.4.

RETIRED-COUPLE BUDGETS

Another way of illustrating the effects of price changes on the cost of living for the elderly is to calculate budgets for retired couples. Household budgets are used frequently by social scientists to compare living costs of different types of families, different areas, racial groups, or age groups. Changes in specified budgets for retired families indicate income adjustments required to maintain a particular standard of living. The first such budget for elderly households was developed by the Social Security Administration in the mid-1940s and was priced by the Bureau of Labor Statistics for thirteen large cities. Similar budgets were derived for 1946, 1947, and 1949. The base was expanded to thirty-four cities in 1950 before this budget was discontinued, because the expenditure and consumption data on which it was based were deemed outdated. In 1959 a revised interim budget for a retired couple was published for twenty larger cities.

In 1967 the Bureau of Labor Statistics began constructing three budgets for a retired couple. These budgets represent the costs of hypothetical lists of goods and services selected in the mid-1960s to be consistent with a high, intermediate, and low standard of living in retirement. The budgets measured the income required to purchase the quantity and quality of goods and services consistent with these standards of living. The budgets assumed that the retired couple participated in normal social community activities and maintained good health and general well-being. Within this framework, three different budgets were designed, each providing a different quantity and quality of goods and services.

The lower-level budget represents a couple that relied mostly on public

TABLE 3.3. Total Personal Consumption Expenditures and Percentage Devoted to Selected Components, 1967–82

Year	Total Expenditures Billions of Dollars	Food and Tobacco Billions of Dollars	Food and Tobacco Percent	Housing and Household Operations Billions of Dollars	Housing and Household Operations Percent	Medical Care Billions of Dollars	Medical Care Percent	Transportation Billions of Dollars	Transportation Percent	Clothing Billions of Dollars	Clothing Percent	All Other Billions of Dollars	All Other Percent
1967	490	119	24.3	144	29.4	35	7.1	63	12.9	46	9.4	83	16.9
1968	537	128	23.8	155	28.9	39	7.3	73	13.6	51	9.5	91	16.9
1969	582	137	23.5	167	28.7	45	7.7	79	13.6	54	9.3	100	17.2
1970	622	150	24.1	178	28.6	50	8.1	81	13.0	56	9.0	107	17.2
1971	672	156	23.2	192	28.6	56	8.3	94	14.0	60	8.9	114	17.0
1972	737	167	22.7	211	28.6	62	8.4	105	14.3	65	8.8	127	17.2
1973	812	185	22.8	233	28.7	69	8.5	115	14.1	72	8.9	138	17.0
1974	888	208	23.4	259	29.2	77	8.7	118	13.3	76	8.5	150	16.9
1975	976	228	23.4	283	29.0	88	9.0	129	13.2	82	8.4	166	17.0
1976	1,084	247	22.8	315	29.1	98	9.0	155	14.3	89	8.2	180	16.6
1977	1,204	266	22.1	352	29.2	113	9.4	179	14.9	97	8.0	197	16.4
1978	1,346	294	21.8	394	29.3	126	9.4	198	14.7	108	8.0	226	16.8
1979	1,507	331	22.0	444	29.5	144	9.5	219	14.5	116	7.7	253	16.8
1980	1,668	366	22.0	496	29.7	167	10.0	237	14.2	124	7.4	278	16.7
1981	1,857	399	21.5	558	30.0	197	10.6	262	14.1	137	7.4	304	16.4
1982	1,992	422	21.2	606	30.4	221	11.1	270	13.5	141	7.1	332	16.7

Sources: Data for 1967–75 obtained from U.S. Department of Commerce, Bureau of Economic Analysis, *The National Income and Production Amounts of the United States, 1929–76 Statistical Tables,* September 1981. Data for 1976–78 obtained from U.S. Department of Commerce, Bureau of Economic Analysis, *Survey of Current Business,* July 1982, vol. 62, no. 7. Data for 1979–82 obtained from U.S. Department of Commerce, Bureau of Economic Analysis, *Survey of Current Business,* July 1983, vol. 63, no. 7.

TABLE 3.4. Implicit Personal Consumption Expenditures Index, 1967–82

Year	Index	Year	Index
1967	81.4	1975	125.2
1968	84.6	1976	131.7
1969	88.4	1977	139.3
1970	92.5	1978	149.1
1971	96.5	1979	162.5
1972	100.0	1980	179.0
1973	105.7	1981	194.1
1974	116.3	1982	205.3

Sources: Data for 1967–75 obtained from U.S. Department of Commerce, Bureau of Economic Analysis, *The National Income and Product Amounts of the United States, 1929–76 Statistical Tables,* September 1981. Data for 1976–78 obtained from U.S. Department of Commerce, Bureau of Economic Analysis, *Survey of Current Business,* July 1982, vol. 62, no. 7. Data for 1979–82 obtained from U.S. Department of Commerce, Bureau of Economic Analysis, *Survey of Current Business,* July 1983, vol. 63, no. 7.

transportation, with the occasional use of an older car to supplement public transportation. Also, the couple is assumed to perform more services for themselves than did those at intermediate- or higher-level budgets. Furthermore, it is assumed that they utilize free community resources for recreation. The intermediate budget included some new car ownership, more paid-for services, and more household appliances and equipment relative to the low budget. Income taxes were included in their budget, since it was assumed that income was not derived from tax-free sources. The higher-level budget was based on a more liberal food budget and a greater quantity and quality of other goods and services.

Composition of the budgets was based on spending decisions reflected in the 1960–61 Consumer Expenditure Survey and other relevant information. Nutritional and health standards determined by scientists and technicians were used in deriving the budgets for the food-at-home and housing components. Related consumption studies were used to determine the quantity and quality of specific items. Surveys of consumer expenditures were also used to provide the selection of food and housing arrangements from the standards determined above. Other expenditure categories include transportation, clothing and personal care, and other consumption items.

The budget share allowances in 1967 for each category, compared to the average consumption pattern for retired couples in the 1960–61 Consumer Expenditure Survey, are shown in Table 3.5. The budgets were updated in August of each year through 1980 by the U.S. Department of Labor's Bureau of Labor Statistics. Each year's changes in prices and tax payments were taken into account. The costs of the budgets were recalculated by incorporating changes in components of the consumer price index to the base-year budget level for these items. (For a more detailed discussion of the development of the retired couples' budgets, see U.S. Bureau of Labor Statistics,

TABLE 3.5. Comparison of Actual Spending Patterns (1960–61) and
1967 Budget Allowances

| Components | Consumption, 1960–61 CES | 1967 Budget Allowance | | |
		Lower Budget	Intermediate Budget	Higher Budget
Total spending	$3,323	$2,556	$3,626	$5,335
Percent				
Total	100%	100%	100%	100%
Food	26	31	29	24
Housing	33	37	37	39
Transportation	9	7	10	13
Clothing and personal care	12	8	10	10
Medical care	11	12	8	6
Other	9	5	6	8

Source: U.S. Bureau of Labor Statistics, *Three Budgets for a Retired Couple in Urban Areas of the United States, 1967–68,* Bulletin no. 1570-6, Washington, D.C.: Government Printing Office, May 1970.

1970.) Later in this chapter, the trends in the budgets for a retired couple are compared to increases in price indexes.

Changes in procedures used to calculate these types of budgets have been recommended by a study panel (Watts, 1980). The panel recommended that four budget levels based on median expenditures obtained from the new continuous Consumer Expenditure Survey be utilized. The reference family for such calculations would be two parents and two children. Median expenditures of reference families would be used for determining the prevailing family standard budget. There would also be three alternative budget levels. The social minimum standard would be half the prevailing family standard. The lower living standard, somewhat analogous to the current lower budget, would be set at two-thirds the prevailing family standard. The social abundance standard would be 50 percent above the prevailing family standard. The 1979 values of these standards for a two-member aged household were $4,919, $6,559, $9,839, and $14,758.

COMPARISONS OF THE CPI, THE PCE, AND FAMILY BUDGET DATA

We have noted how the CPI, the PCE, and family budgets differ in measurement, calculation, and estimates of changes in the cost of living. While the broadest CPI covers only expenditures by urban consumers, the PCE covers all expenditures of households and nonprofit organizations. The retired-couple budgets indicate the income typically used each year to maintain low, intermediate, and high levels of living. Thus, these three measures would be expected to reflect different rates of change during recent years.

The CPI indicates an increase of 147 percent in prices from 1967 to 1980, whereas the PCE indicates an increase of 120 percent over the same period. As expected, the latter change is smaller than the increase in prices given by the CPI. The family budget data indicate that the income required for the low budget in 1967 was $2,671 compared to $6,644 in 1980, indicating that the low-income elderly couple required 149 percent more income in 1980 to maintain the same living standard as in 1967. The intermediate budget went from $3,857 in 1967 to $9,434 in 1980, an increase of 145 percent. The high-level budget required $13,923 in 1980 to maintain the living level obtained in 1967 for $6,049, an increase of 131 percent. The income required to maintain a constant standard of living as indicated by the lower budget rose by a rate greater than increases of either price index, whereas the intermediate and higher budgets rose slightly less than the CPI.

One of the major differences in the PCE and CPI price indexes has been their treatment of housing (Blinder, 1980). Before January 1983 the CPI included cost of houses, mortgage interest, insurance, taxes, and repairs. The CPI's treatment of housing and mortgage rates drew considerable attention during the late 1970s and early 1980s. Historically the index used current house prices and current mortgage rates. A weight based on 1972–73 information about home purchases was used in calculating the housing component. If a family purchased a house during the base period, the total purchase price was counted as a current expenditure in the survey of consumption expenditures, and the interest cost of the mortgage financing over the first half of its life was also counted as a current expenditure. This treatment was criticized because it treated housing as a current consumer outlay and ignored the fact that housing is an investment that provides services over a number of years. An alternative is to use a rental equivalent method to measure home ownership costs. This is the method used in calculating the PCE index. Further details on this adjustment are provided by Gillingham and Lane (1982). As of January 1983, the Bureau of Labor Statistics adopted the procedure for the CPI for all urban consumers. In January 1985 the same modifications will be incorporated into the CPI for wage earners and clerical workers.

Since housing accounts for a large part of a family's expenditures, different treatments of housing expenditures have influenced the PCE's and CPI's estimates of inflation over most of the years examined in this study. The effect of the different measures of housing from 1972 to 1982 has been examined by Bunn and Triplett (1983), who calculated that the difference in the treatment of housing in the CPI and the PCE between 1972 and 1982 accounted for approximately two-thirds of the cumulative difference between the two measures during this period.

All components of the CPI did not experience the same rate of change during the years for which trends in real income and expenditures are examined in other chapters. For the CPI, Tables 3.1 and 3.2 indicate that the compo-

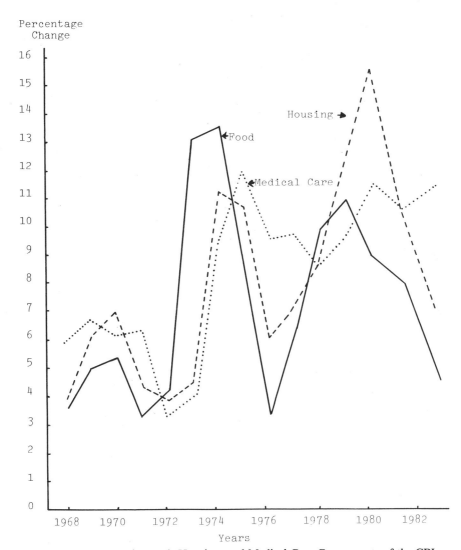

FIGURE 3.1. Change in Food, Housing, and Medical Care Components of the CPI, 1967–82
Source: Bureau of Labor Statistics, *Monthly Labor Review,* March 1983, Table 18.

nent differing the most from the overall annual price increase was food. The year-to-year changes for food, housing, and medical care are illustrated in Figure 3.1. From 1967 to 1977 the annual rate of increase in food prices fluctuated from 3.1 percent in 1971 and 1976 to around 13 percent in 1972 and 1973. If food prices increased 13 percent and all other items increased only 6.2 percent (1973), people were likely to have substituted away from food to relatively cheaper products or from more expensive food to less expensive food, implying a changing distribution of consumption. There are other years in which food prices increased relatively faster than all other prices, but in some years the opposite occurred. The proportion of total consumption expenditures allocated to food decreased from 24.3 percent in 1967 to 21.2 percent in 1982 (see Table 3.3). Between 1972 and 1975, expenditures on food increased relative to other items before beginning to decline again. In the retired-couple budgets, the proportion of the different budgets devoted to food increased over this period. Food was 29.5 percent of the low budget in 1967 and remained near this level until substantial food price increases in 1972. From 1973 to 1980, food expenditures represented approximately 31 percent of this budget. The same pattern is observed for the intermediate and high budgets.

The housing and medical components of retired-couple budgets can be compared in the same way to see the effect of the relative price differences. Housing and medical price increases also fluctuated substantially during the 1970s. These changes in relative prices altered the budget shares in the retired-family budgets. All three budgets for a retired couple showed substantial increases in the proportions for health expenditures between 1967 and 1980. The changes in budget shares were especially large during the last three or four years. Proportions allocated to housing in 1980 were slightly lower than in 1967 for the low- and intermediate-level budgets. For the high budget, the 1980 housing proportion was slightly larger than it was in 1967.

Aggregate personal consumption expenditures in Table 3.3 indicate that U.S. households were allocating larger proportions of their budgets to housing and health items in the late 1970s and early 1980s than they were a decade earlier. The share going to transportation was also larger in the late 1970s than it was in the late 1960s, but it decreased in the last three or four years. On the other hand, the proportion spent for clothing decreased continuously between 1967 and 1982.

CONSUMER PRICE INDEXES FOR THE ELDERLY

Several researchers have attempted to construct a price index specifically for older persons. Using seven weights derived from the 1972–73 Consumer Expenditure Survey, Bridges and Packard (1981) constructed a CPI for older persons (CPI-O) and compared it to a modified CPI for urban wage earners and clerical workers (CPI-W). The weights used in the construction of this index are shown in Table 3.6, and the trends in these indexes are reported in Table 3.7.

During the period 1967–79, the CPI-O increased from 100.0 to 219.9, while the CPI-W rose from 100.0 to 217.7. Table 3.7 shows that the CPI-O typically rose by a slightly higher percentage than the CPI-W, but the total

TABLE 3.6. Distribution of Costs of Constructed CPI Market Baskets, by Expenditure Class

Expenditure Class	CPI-O (Percentage)	CPI-W (Percentage)
All classes	100.0	100.0
Food and beverages	21.6	20.0
Housing	38.5	39.1
Apparel and upkeep	5.9	7.2
Transportation	15.8	20.9
Medical care	9.5	4.0
Entertainment	4.2	4.3
Other goods and services	4.5	4.5

Source: Benjamin Bridges and Michael Packard, "Price and Income Changes for the Elderly," *Social Security Bulletin* 44 (1), January 1981, p. 5.

Note: Quantities or market baskets for 1972–73 at 1967 prices.

TABLE 3.7. Constructed Consumer Price Indexes: Annual Indexes and Percentage Changes, 1967–79 (1967 = 100)

Year	CPI-O Index	CPI-O Percentage Change	CPI-W Index	CPI-W Percentage Change
1967	100.0	—	100.0	—
1968	104.2	4.2	104.2	4.2
1969	109.9	5.5	109.9	5.5
1970	116.5	6.0	116.2	5.7
1971	121.7	4.5	121.2	4.3
1972	125.7	3.3	125.1	3.2
1973	133.1	5.9	132.3	5.8
1974	147.9	11.1	147.0	11.1
1975	162.0	9.5	160.7	9.3
1976	172.0	6.2	170.6	6.2
1977	183.5	6.7	181.7	6.5
1978	197.6	7.7	195.2	7.4
1979	219.9	11.3	217.7	11.5

Source: Benjamin Bridges and Michael Packard, "Price and Income Changes for the Elderly," *Social Security Bulletin* 44 (1), January 1981, p. 4.

difference over the twelve years was less than 2 percent of the total increase. The higher rate of increase in the CPI-O is the result of the elderly spending larger shares of their income on medical care and food. Between 1967 and 1979 the prices of these items increased by the greatest percentage (see Table 3.1). The greater expenditure by older persons on medical care combined with the fact that the price increases in health services were greater than increases in any other group accounted for half the difference between the growth rate of the two CPIs.

Borzilleri (1978) also constructed a CPI for older persons for January 1970 through March 1977 employing fifteen expenditure weights based on the 1972–73 Consumer Expenditure Survey. His estimates differ from those of Bridges and Packard in the treatment of housing. Borzilleri also constructed a modified CPI for all consumers using the same concept of housing. His CPI-O rises more rapidly than that of Bridges and Packard between 1970 and 1978, whereas his revised CPI for all consumers increases at approximately the same rate as that shown in Table 3.7. The Borzilleri CPI-O rose 48.8 percent during the period, compared to 46.9 percent for his modified CPI for all consumers; that is, his CPI-O rose by 1.04 percent for each percentage increase in the modified CPI.

Bridges and Packard reviewed several other indexes of prices for older persons and found that these indexes increased slightly faster than their own CPI-O. In summary, their evidence suggests that consumer price increases on the goods and services purchased by the elderly rose at a slightly greater rate than those for the entire population until the late 1970s (also see Boskin and Hurd, 1982). This trend may have been reversed in the last few years. Grimaldi (1982) estimates that prices rose faster for the elderly in 1973–74, at essentially the same rate for all households between 1975 and 1978, and at a slower rate for the elderly from 1978 to 1981. As a result, the average inflation rate for all households was 9.2 percent between 1973 and 1981 but only 8.8 percent for aged households.

Even if the index of prices faced by the average older person rises at a rate different from that of the general index, it still may be desirable to use the CPI-W to determine changes in real income of the elderly. Michael (1979) supported this conclusion by showing greater variations in the rate of increase in prices within age groups than between them. He employed the 1960–61 Consumer Expenditure Survey and constructed a price index that he called an expenditure price index (EPI). The EPI excluded house purchases and employed fixed expenditure weights. The sample means for seven age groups suggested a higher rate of inflation for older persons, but regression analysis suggested that no groups consistently experienced higher rates of inflation. Michael concluded by arguing that "two or two hundred, such indices may not be more adequate than one CPI if the within-group dispersion among households is larger relative to the between group means, and especially so if there is little correlation over time in the groups' relative changes in the price indices" (Michael, 1979, p. 34).

Barnes and Zedlewski (1981) estimated that changes in relative prices from 1974 to 1980 had only small effects on budget allocations of elderly households. This is based on their finding that food, fuel, and shelter expenditures (for renters) were relatively unresponsive to geographical price differences reflected by interregional indexes. Medical care and all other expenditures were more responsive.

While the CPI is used in most of the analysis throughout this book because it is widely used in indexing transfer payments, it probably overestimates the price increases for the elderly during the period of analysis, so trends in real income will be understated. Data from this chapter are used for indexing or deflating nominal income and expenditures discussed in other parts of this book.

4 Income Patterns of Older Persons

It is widely believed that because the elderly live on fixed incomes, their real income declines in the presence of inflation. This chapter examines the life-cycle pattern of income of older persons and the experience of the 1970s. The analysis of income changes uses two distinct methods of identifying changes in the well-being of older persons. The first method is to examine a specific set of individuals born within a few years of each other. This analysis was done using longitudinal surveys such as the RHS and PSID. Such a group of individuals is called a cohort, and the cohort analysis presented below will indicate how the income of these individuals changed over time. The second method of analysis is to examine year-to-year changes in the income of a particular age group such as persons aged 55 to 64 or 65 years and older. The composition of an age group changes as new people enter and others age out of the group. Thus some of the observed changes for an age group are attributable to the different life experiences of its new and old members. The advantage of using the age group method of comparison is that it holds constant age or the stage of life, such as retirement. The advantage of the cohort analysis is that the composition of the group is constant except for the death of some of the individuals. Both methods provide useful information concerning the trend in well-being of the elderly.

INCOME OF THE RETIREMENT HISTORY STUDY COHORT, 1968-74

The Retirement History Study (RHS) is a series of surveys conducted for the Social Security Administration using respondents aged 58 to 63 in 1969. Married men, nonmarried men, and nonmarried women were interviewed every two years until 1979. At the time of this research, data from 1969 to 1975 were available. A comprehensive list of income, work, and health questions was asked of more than 11,000 respondents. The RHS has become the most widely used data for examining the income and work patterns of older persons (Irelan, 1972).

In each interview, respondents in the RHS were asked detailed questions concerning their cash income in the preceding year. This analysis describes the income of these people in 1968, 1970, 1972, and 1974 by determining their mean income as reported in 1969 to 1975. The trends in average nominal and real income for various demographic groups of interest were examined. Married couples were the basic unit in this analysis, although their income pattern was compared to that of nonmarried men and women. The couples were sorted by age, health status, race, receipt of social security or employer pension benefits, and retirement status.

The sources of income examined were earnings, employer pensions, social security, other governmental cash transfers, and asset income. Earnings are shown separately in Tables 4.1, 4.3, 4.4, 4.5, and 4.6 for husband and wife and represent both wage and self-employment earnings. The "other transfers" income includes income from disability and welfare programs. Asset income is composed of income from rent, stocks and bonds, and savings accounts. All values are reported in current-year nominal dollars except for the row titled "total real income" in the tables.

The sample population of families consisted of all husband-and-wife couples who remained together throughout the survey period; that is, only those couples who were interviewed in every survey year were included in the base sample. Thus, this section is an example of cohort analysis, which follows the same group of individuals over the survey period. The mean for each income source is calculated from the set of respondents that had usable answers to the question concerning the specific income source in question, including zero values. As a result, the number of respondents varies slightly across the income sources in Tables 4.1, 4.3, 4.4, 4.5, and 4.6. This procedure and minor rounding errors are the reasons that the sum of the means by source does not exactly equal the mean total nominal income. The sample size shown at the bottom of each table is the number of observations with complete income data.

All Married Couples

Table 4.1 shows the income history of all husband-wife couples in the Retirement History Study. The husbands in this sample were 57 to 62 years of age in 1968 and thus were 63 to 68 years old by 1974. The mean nominal income of $9,773 in 1968 decreased slightly over the six-year period to $9,129 in 1974. During this period, the consumer price index rose from 104.2 to 147.7. As a result, the real income in 1967 dollars of this sample declined sharply from $9,380 to $6,181 during the six-year period, a fall of 34 percent. Although this was a significant decline in real income during this period, this change was due primarily to life-cycle decisions that result in declining hours of work in old age. We will outline the income changes without attempting to disentangle the direct inflation effects.

The changing composition of income is of particular interest to our study. In 1968, earnings represented 88.2 percent of family income, but by 1974, nominal earnings of the husband had dropped by almost half and family earnings accounted for only 45 percent of total income. The decline in

TABLE 4.1. Mean Income for Couples in Retirement History Study, 1968–74

Source	1968	1970	1972	1974
Sample size	3,361	3,416	3,376	3,725
Earnings				
Husband	$7,066	$6,545	$5,247	$2,938
Wife	1,550	1,546	1,396	1,172
Pension	340	551	1,026	1,709
Social security	190	320	967	2,102
Other transfers	63	220	291	262
Asset income	565	738	937	1,039
Total nominal income	$9,773	$9,762	$9,683	$9,129
Total real income[a]	9,380	8,394	7,728	6,181

Source: Retirement History Study, 1969–75 interviews.
[a] Values in 1967 dollars as measured by the CPI.

mean earnings was the result primarily of fewer hours per worker and fewer persons in the labor force. These are expected life-cycle effects as persons generally reduce their labor supply with age. This pattern of earnings decline was also influenced by changing real wages and family income which may have been altered by inflation. The reduced importance of earnings with age leads some people to conclude that the income of the elderly will not rise in response to higher prices. Thus, it is significant to note that even when the husbands were aged 63 to 68, earnings comprised half the average family income.

Employer pensions and social security benefits accounted for an increasing proportion of average family income as the household aged. Pensions represented 3.5 percent and social security 1.9 percent of family income in 1968 but increased in importance to 18.7 and 23 percent, respectively, in 1974. The growth in mean pension and social security income was primarily in response to an increased number of people receiving these payments. Inflation may have altered pension income by influencing labor supply choices as noted above. In addition, rising consumer prices will have decreased the real benefits unless nominal benefits were raised by a rate equal to the rate of inflation. Chapter 6, which examines the change in nominal and real benefits after a person has begun to receive the pension, provides a more direct assessment of the effects of inflation on current beneficiaries.

The significant rise in mean asset income between 1968 and 1972, while the average age of the sample increased from 60 to 64 years, is consistent with a growth in personal wealth in the years immediately prior to retirement. Hurd and Shoven (1982b) show that the real value of stocks and bonds for RHS couples fell during these years, while the real value of bank accounts rose. Real income from assets depends on the rate of return earned by the asset after subtracting the change in the overall price level. The elderly will experience a greater inflation effect than others only if their investment portfolio differs from the assets of the remainder of the population.

TABLE 4.2. Mean Real Income of Couples in RHS by Personal Characteristics, 1968–74

Characteristic	1968	1970	1972	1974
Age of husband in 1968				
57–58	$ 9,564	$ 8,764	$8,753	$6,966
59–60	9,348	8,370	7,619	5,875
61–62	9,186	7,977	6,589	5,573
Race of husband				
White	9,748	8,676	7,999	6,354
Nonwhite	5,891	5,649	5,114	4,451
Health status of husband[a]				
Excellent health	11,124	10,448	9,701	7,949
Good health	9,688	8,802	7,880	7,395
Moderate health limitation	8,301	5,466	5,075	6,986
Severe health limitation	4,696	4,775	5,161	4,722
Very severe health limitation	4,740	3,987	4,391	3,933
Recipient of social security benefits				
Receiving benefits	6,422	5,911	6,050	5,603
Not receiving benefits	9,884	8,892	8,677	7,220
Nonmarried[b]				
Men	4,846	4,821	4,737	3,917
Women	3,148	3,050	3,045	2,609

Source: Retirement History Study, 1969–75 interviews.

Note: Values are in 1967 dollars as measured by the CPI.

[a] Health was measured by the Duke Health Index with values ranging from 1 for excellent health to 5 for very severe health limitations.

[b] The nonmarried sample was chosen using the same selection requirements used for the married sample.

The smallest category of income was other government transfers, which represented less than 3 percent of income in all years. The effect of inflation on this form of income depends on the government's response to higher prices in the form of increased benefits.

Age and Income Patterns

A comparison of the real income of persons of different ages shows some of the life-cycle effects on real income (see Table 4.2). The sample was divided into two-year age groups. Note that the pattern of real income was generally the same for the three groups but that the oldest group had a consistently lower mean income. The reason is that the older families have substantially lower earnings, especially in the later years. For example, families with husbands aged 63 to 64 in 1974 had total nominal earnings of $6,446, compared with $2,269 for families whose husbands were aged 67 to 68. Large declines in family earnings occurred after the husband passed age 65. For example, the mean earnings of husbands in the oldest cohort dropped from $6,506 in 1970 when these men were aged 63 to 64 to $2,810 in 1972. Similarly, earnings for the middle group declined from $5,307 in 1972, when they were 63 to 64 years of age, to $2,152 in 1974, when the husbands were 65 to 66 years old.

These data reveal other life-cycle changes in the composition of income. Pension and social security benefits represented 56 percent of family income in 1974 for the older group, whereas earnings comprised only 27.6 percent. For the youngest group, earnings were 62.6 percent of total income, and pension and social security benefits accounted for only 26.5 percent. A further indication of these life-cycle differences is that nominal income of the youngest group was higher at the end of the period than in 1968, whereas nominal income was lower for the older groups. As a result, the real income of the youngest group fell by 27 percent between 1968 and 1974, compared with a decline of more than 37 percent for the older groups. These comparisons, along with an examination of income changes over time, clearly indicate life-cycle effects of earnings for families with husbands in their late fifties and sixties. Any assessment of the inflation effect on family income must be made with care so as not to confound these effects.

These results can be compared with those of Hurd and Shoven (1982b), who found smaller declines in mean real income for RHS when nominal income was deflated by a modified CPI for older persons. Their findings were due to the inclusion of the value of housing, medicare, and medicaid in their calculations. Also see Barnes and Zedlewski (1981) for an examination of the RHS income data.

Racial Differences in Income

The average income of nonwhites was significantly lower than that of white families in each year. The mean income of nonwhites ranged between 60 and 70 percent of the average income for white couples. The racial differences are primarily due to the substantially lower earnings of nonwhite husbands. The lower wealth of nonwhites is illustrated by their asset income, which was less than one-quarter of the return to assets for whites in every year except 1974. In addition, the pension benefits of nonwhites were only about half those received by white families. Benefits from other government transfer income were comparable for the two groups. Both groups exhibited the same pattern of relatively constant nominal income and declining real income between 1968 and 1974. The fall in real income over the period was only 24 percent for nonwhites, compared to 35 percent for whites.

Health Status and Income of the Elderly

The health status of older persons influences their income levels and also the sources of their income. Table 4.2 shows the mean real income of the RHS cohort depending on the health of the husband as measured by his ranking on the Duke Health Index (Fillenbaum and Maddox, 1977). Health status declines as the index falls from one to five. The samples in each health group in each year are based on the current health of the individual, and therefore the number of persons in each category varies across the survey years. Notice that total income fell as health declined in each survey year. Earnings were a less important component of income for those with health limitations; other government transfers such as disability and welfare were considerably more important. The decline in real income for those in poor health was less than the decline for those that remained in good health, because a larger proportion of the income for those in poor health came from government programs that were directly or implicitly indexed. In addition, persons with health limitations were typically already out of the labor force and thus did not have large declines in earnings with age as did those who remained in good health.

Acceptance of Social Security and Private Pension Benefits

Significant differences in income were observed when the mean income of families with social security benefits was compared to that of those who were not currently receiving these payments. First, mean incomes were over 22 percent higher for families not receiving social security benefits. As one would expect, earnings of the husbands were substantially greater when there was no social security income. For families receiving social security payments, these benefits represented as much as 38 percent of average income in 1974. Pension income was also greater for families drawing social security income. These observations are to be expected and reflect life-cycle labor supply decisions. Older persons reduce their hours of work or withdraw from the labor force, which tends to reduce their earnings and increase pension and social security benefits. The income data over the sample period should be compared with care, since the number of families receiving benefits rises as the sample population ages. It is interesting to note, however, that the decline in real income was substantially less for those receiving social security benefits.

Sorting of the sample by receipt of employer pension benefits revealed a similar pattern. The average pension benefit for those currently receiving this income rose from $2,513 in 1968 to $3,588 in 1974. Pension income represented over 34 percent of family income for recipients in 1974 and, combined with social security payments, accounted for 60 percent of family income. As expected, those with no pension income had larger earnings in each of the survey years. For both recipients and nonrecipients of social security and pension benefits, real income declined during the survey period.

Marital Status

The RHS sample also contained nonmarried men and women who were aged 58 to 63 in 1969. The sample consisted of all nonmarried men and women in the survey for each year. The mean real income of these groups, shown in Table 4.2, can be compared with income patterns of couples shown

TABLE 4.3. Mean Income for Families Whose Husbands Retired Between 1969 and 1971

Source	1968	1970	1972	1974
Sample size	494	445	502	504
Earnings				
Husband	$ 8,059	$4,091	$ 959	$ 287
Wife	1,433	1,341	1,035	986
Pension	160	1,171	1,714	2,147
Social security	92	832	1,753	2,751
Other transfers	33	400	309	313
Asset income	685	842	1,165	1,309
Total nominal income	$10,458	$8,470	$6,552	$7,612
Total real income[a]	10,036	7,283	5,229	5,154

Source: Retirement History Study, 1969–75 interviews.
Note: Husband was in the labor force in 1969 but not in the survey years of 1971, 1973, and 1975.
[a] Values in 1967 dollars as measured by the CPI.

in Table 4.1. The principal observation is that the average income of nonmarried men was 52 to 63 percent of the income of couples, while the income of single women was only 34 to 42 percent of couples' incomes during this period. The income of single persons relative to couples rose slightly between 1968 and 1974. The changing income pattern observed for the couples is also apparent for the nonmarried individuals; earnings declined in importance, while pensions and social security provided an increasing proportion of total income.

Retirement and Income in Old Age

People tend to reduce their hours of work as they age. Many workers abruptly change their work life by going from full-time work to complete retirement; others switch to part-time jobs, reducing the number of hours of work per week. These life-cycle changes will lower annual earnings, and because retirement benefits rarely are equal to preretirement earnings, annual income tends to fall with age. Thus, much of the decline in mean income observed for the RHS cohort is an expected life-cycle pattern that follows from declines in the average work effort of the individuals.

To illustrate further the effect of retirement on the income of older families, the RHS sample of couples was divided into four groups by the retirement date of the husband (see Tables 4.3, 4.4, 4.5, and 4.6). The four groups are: (1) husbands who worked in 1969 but were not in the labor force in the other survey years of 1971, 1973, and 1975; (2) husbands who worked in 1969 and 1971 but not in 1973 and 1975; (3) husbands who worked in 1969, 1971, and 1973 but not in 1975; and (4) husbands who worked in all survey years.

The income data were for the year prior to the interview date when the husband was reported to be in or out of the labor force. In each of the first

TABLE 4.4. Mean Income for Families Whose Husbands Retired Between 1971 and 1973

Source	1968	1970	1972	1974
Sample size	749	751	764	765
Earnings				
Husband	$ 8,076	$ 9,012	$4,490	$ 199
Wife	1,600	1,659	1,402	1,016
Pension	142	210	1,479	2,659
Social security	56	125	1,195	2,936
Other transfers	20	93	390	298
Asset income	489	681	933	985
Total nominal income	$10,372	$11,623	$9,663	$7,868
Total real income[a]	9,953	9,994	7,712	5,327

Source: Retirement History Study, 1969–75 interviews.
Note: Husband was in the labor force in 1969 and 1971 but not in the survey years of 1973 and 1975.
[a] Values in 1967 dollars as measured by the CPI.

TABLE 4.5. Mean Income for Families Whose Husbands Retired Between 1973 and 1975

Source	1968	1970	1972	1974
Sample size	580	577	579	579
Earnings				
Husband	$ 8,043	$ 8,721	$ 9,344	$ 4,108
Wife	1,625	1,742	1,661	1,409
Pension	208	204	282	1,937
Social security	39	66	341	2,073
Other transfers	107	61	110	171
Asset income	370	462	565	820
Total nominal income	$10,391	$11,167	$12,222	$10,414
Total real income[a]	9,972	9,602	9,754	7,051

Source: Retirement History Study, 1969–75 interviews.
Note: Husband was in the labor force in 1969, 1971, and 1973 but not in the survey year of 1975.
[a] Values in 1967 dollars as measured by the CPI.

three groups, earnings dropped by approximately one-half in the year between interviews where the husband first was working and then retired; for example, 1972 for Group 2 (see Table 4.4). Tables 4.3 and 4.4 show that earnings of the husband were trivial in the postretirement years and Tables 4.4, 4.5, and 4.6 indicate that prior to retirement earnings continued to rise. Of particular interest is the finding that real income prior to retirement either rose or fell only slightly. Real income of a cohort after retirement also did not decline much; compare 1972 with 1974 in Table 4.3. This suggests that much of the decline in real income shown in Tables 4.1 and 4.2 was due to labor supply decisions as families shifted from work to retirement. As older persons retired, their earnings fell and pensions and social security benefits rose.

TABLE 4.6. Mean Income for Families Whose Husbands Remained in the Labor Force from 1969 to 1975.

Source	1968	1970	1972	1974
Sample size	743	745	736	737
Earnings				
Husband	$ 8,155	$ 8,741	$ 9,261	$ 9,082
Wife	1,626	1,756	1,686	1,552
Pension	117	194	282	643
Social security	36	84	316	966
Other transfers	17	45	64	70
Asset income	449	622	707	943
Total nominal income	$10,399	$11,294	$12,176	$13,298
Total real income[a]	9,980	9,711	9,718	9,003

Source: Retirement History Study, 1969–75 interviews.
[a] Values in 1967 dollars as measured by the CPI.

Typically these payments were less than preretirement earnings, and so incomes were lower in the retirement years. This pattern is observed for all demographic groups. In the following chapters, we will isolate these life-cycle choices from direct inflation effects by focusing on the different sources of income.

PANEL STUDY OF INCOME DYNAMICS, 1968–76

The Panel Study of Income Dynamics (PSID) is a longitudinal survey of approximately 5,000 households begun in 1968 by the Survey Research Center of the University of Michigan. The same families were reinterviewed throughout the period. This analysis, performed by Mary Jane Gorman, employs 865 households whose head was age 55 or older in 1968. Institutionalized older persons and noninstitutionalized elderly who neither maintained a separate household nor were designated head when living with relatives were excluded from the sample. This survey is quite useful in that it includes nine years of data on the sample population. Its major shortcoming is the small sample size of older households. Like the preceding discussion of the RHS respondents, this examination is an example of cohort analysis, which follows a group of individuals over time as they age and respond to changing economic conditions.

Trends in family income for a household whose head was 55 years or older are shown in Table 4.7. Nominal income rose from $7,002 in 1967 to $9,230 in 1975, an increase of 31.8 percent. During the same period, the consumer price index rose by over 61 percent, producing a decline in real income to $5,726. This decline is similar to that observed in the RHS cohort. The composition of income also changed as the sample population aged. Earnings declined from 63 percent of total income in 1967 to 30 percent in 1975, while

TABLE 4.7. Mean Family Income with Head 55 Years or Older
in the PSID, by Source

Source	1967	1969	1971	1973	1975
Earnings[a]	$4,444	$4,277	$3,855	$3,213	$2,732
Transfers[b]	1,191[c]	1,505	2,082	2,875	3,809
Asset income[d]	1,009	1,303	1,351	1,443	1,901
Income of others in household[e]	357[f]	548	726	869	789
Total nominal income	$7,002	$7,633	$8,014	$8,401	$9,230
Total real income[g]	7,002	6,952	6,607	6,312	5,726

Source: Data derived from information provided by Mary Jane Gorman, who used information from the Panel Study of Income Dynamics.

[a] Labor part of farm income and business income, wages of head and wife, bonuses, overtime, commissions, professional practice, labor part of income from roomers and boarders.

[b] ADC, AFDC, social security, retirement income, annuities and pensions, unemployment and workmen's compensation, alimony and child support, income from relatives, wife's transfer income, other income not included elsewhere.

[c] Includes transfer income of all members of the household.

[d] Asset part of income from farm, business, roomers, etc.; income from rent, interest and dividends; and wife's asset income.

[e] Taxable and transfer income of persons in household other than head or wife.

[f] Includes only taxable income of others in household.

[g] Values in 1967 dollars.

transfers and asset income increased from 17 and 14 percent to 41 and 21 percent of the total income. These changes occurred in large part in response to life-cycle allocation of labor supply and reflect declining labor supply and increased likelihood of pension acceptance. By contrast, the nominal income of younger households in the PSID rose by 96 percent, implying an increase in real income of 21 percent.

The effect of inflation on the well-being of the elderly can be examined further by applying regression analysis to the PSID data. The trend in the economic well-being of older persons was estimated by comparing total household income to the retired-couple's budget (see Chapter 3) as the families aged over the nine-year survey period. In general, the value of the budget rises to keep a family at the same level of consumption over time.

In these regressions, the dependent variable is the ratio of total household income to the retired-couple's budget adjusted for family size and place of residence. The regressions hold constant factors contributing to different levels of income across the sample. Thus, the regression variables indicating year effects measure the change in real income of the sample over the period. It is important to note that the retirement variable will capture most of the life-cycle effect of reduced labor supply shown in the trends in mean income reported earlier in this chapter. This variable has a substantial negative effect on real income for families with husbands between the ages of 60 and 64 and 65 and 69.

The model was estimated for age subsamples based on husbands aged 60 to 64, 65 to 69, and 70 to 75 in 1968. For each age sample, only those households in which the head did not change during the survey period were included in the sample. There is no evidence that there was a significant difference in economic well-being in any survey year (1968–75) relative to 1967. The sample groups included households at all levels of economic well-being, from upper-income to poor families. Previous analysis indicated that the high- and low-income families depended on different sources of income. Although, on average, no significant difference in real income was evident as households aged from 1967 to 1975, the income of one group may have been improving while that of the other was declining.

The same model was tested for two income groups, those with incomes greater than or equal to the intermediate-level budget in 1967 and those with 1967 incomes less than the 1967 budget. For those with the higher real income in 1967, all year effects were negative, although not significantly different from 1967. For the poor households, real income was significantly higher in all reported years relative to 1967. The largest and most significant effect was for 1972, a year of suppressed measured inflation under the influence of wage and price controls. Even in the subsequent high inflation years that followed, however, the economic position of these elderly households was improved over earlier years. The magnitude of these year effects indicated a slight decline in real income after 1972. The real income of the higher-income group may have declined slightly over the nine-year period. Although those households with income initially below the intermediate budget requirement were, on average, more successful than households with higher incomes in maintaining or improving their economic positions, the poorer households remained in a much worse position overall.

The income pattern of the PSID respondents was similar to that of the RHS cohort. As these cohorts aged, their real income declined, but this was due primarily to reductions in hours of work. Controlling for retirement, both groups had relatively constant real income before retirement, declines at retirement, and then constant real incomes during retirement years. It is also apparent that lower-income persons whose income was derived primarily from government transfers were the least vulnerable to declines in real income with inflation.

CONSUMER EXPENDITURE SURVEY, 1972–73

In 1972–73 the Consumer Expenditure Survey (CES) was conducted by the Bureau of Labor Statistics to obtain information for updating the consumer price index. The survey consisted of two separate parts: (1) a diary portion in which respondents kept a record of selected expenditures for two one-week periods, and (2) an interview panel, in which families reported information every three months. The interview component covered the years 1972 and

TABLE 4.8. Source of Income by Age of Household Head, 1972–73 CES

Source	Age of Household Head	
	Less Than 55 Years	55 and Older
Earnings	$10,692.19	$4,734.30
Social security and pension benefits	355.40	2,137.49
Self-employment	934.00	771.39
Dividends and interest	176.14	830.02
Rents	75.68	200.75
Welfare and public assistance	118.54	87.44
Regular contributions for support	96.34	24.49
Other	358.43	180.43
Totals	$12,806.72	$8,966.31

Source: Calculated from data in *Consumer Expenditure Survey Series, Interview Survey, 1972–73,* U.S. Department of Labor, Report No. 455-4, 1977, table 5.

1973, with each year including approximately 10,000 different families. Approximately 3,600 of the families each year had a head of household 55 years of age and older, which is the age group of special interest in this study. The CES was treated as two cross-sectional surveys, and the results from 1972 were compared with those for 1973. This comparison showed the change in income for a large sample of older persons between 1972 and 1973. The CES differs from the RHS and the PSID in that the 1973 sample does not include the same people that were interviewed in 1972. In this analysis, we examine the income of groups of similar ages in the two survey years, for example, persons aged 60 to 64 in 1972 to persons aged 60 to 64 in 1973.

In the following discussion, we make some comparisons of income patterns of the 55-and-older group to all other households. Then we make a detailed examination of income data for several subsamples of elderly households in 1972 and 1973. Since both years were parts of the same survey, most Bureau of Labor Statistics tabulations combine the two years' data. For our study, there is special interest in the differences between the two years, in order to see how increases in prices may have influenced household decisions. Even though these contrasts involve households with similar characteristics, they are not the same groups of households each year. Unless specifically noted, "household" refers both to families and to unrelated individuals.

Differences in Income by Age

Some general differences in sources and levels of income for those 55 and over relative to the rest of the population are evident from published data for the combined years 1972–73 (see Table 4.8). Total income for elderly households averaged around 70 percent of that for younger households, but per capita income was slightly higher for the 55-and-over group because of a difference in average household size. Households with a head 55 years of age or older had an average of 1.98 persons per household, whereas the younger group averaged 3.38 persons. This comparison may be misleading for two reasons, however. First, the older group consisted primarily of adults, and second, using 55 years of age as a classification point means that the older group included a number of households with members still active in the work force. Consequently, the numbers do not accurately reflect income levels of the older component of the population which was retired. These issues are pursued in later discussions of tabulations for various subgroups of the elderly.

Differences in the amounts of income received from various sources by households with a head aged 55 and older as compared with households that have younger heads provide some information about the impact of price changes. For example, the ways in which wages and retirement benefits adjusted in response to inflation had significantly different effects on younger and older households. Wage rate adjustments remained important for elderly households, however, since more than 50 percent of their income came from earnings in the labor market.

There was not as much difference between the two age groups in the amounts of self-employment income as there were in some of the other sources of income. One area for which there was a sizable difference was the proportion of income from capital assets. Around 11.5 percent of the older group's income was obtained from dividends, interest, and rents, compared with only 2 percent for the younger group. The extent to which unanticipated inflation influenced the value of capital assets can therefore have a significant differential effect on the resulting income streams of various segments of the population. The three other components, welfare, public assistance, regular contributions from outside the consumer unit, and all other sources of income were relatively insignificant for each group of households but considerably smaller in absolute levels for the older segment. Although the latter sources of income undoubtedly were very important for some individual elderly households, they were not very large in the overall picture.

Age Differences in the Older Population

When households of the elderly were subdivided into five age groups, each group indicated an increase in total nominal income between 1972 and 1973 (see Table 4.9). The percentage increases varied from 11.6 for the 60–64 age group to 17.4 for the 70–74 age group. All the increases were greater than the increase of 6.2 percent in the consumer price index between 1972 and 1973, so real income for each age group of older persons rose. The relative increases in per capita income were slightly less, since the 1973 group of households averaged 1.5 percent more individuals than the 1972 sample.

Increases were observed in most sources of income between 1972 and 1973. Retirement benefits, dividends and interest, and other income sources increased for each age group. Three of the five age groups had a decrease in

TABLE 4.9. Average Income by Age of Household Head for Those 55 Years of Age and Older, 1972–73 CES

	Age of Household Head				
Source	55–59	60–64	65–69	70–74	75 +
1972					
Wages	$ 9,717.83	$ 6,729.64	$2,752.82	$ 946.94	$ 570.56
Social security and pensions	612.40	1,242.80	2,810.75	2,923.33	2,624.94
Self-employment	1,141.73	1,164.38	565.73	266.29	253.38
Dividends and interest	475.17	722.25	827.54	858.42	774.92
Rents	198.81	180.35	105.78	163.28	273.92
Unemployment	109.51	82.83	51.31	25.58	52.16
Welfare, public assistance	65.78	99.48	91.58	117.56	130.51
Other sources	170.30	131.41	82.40	33.61	45.46
Total income	$12,491.52	$10,353.13	$7,287.91	$5,335.01	$4,725.86
1973					
Wages	$10,783.20	$ 38.54	$2,686.21	$1,404.51	$ 608.44
Social security and pensions	787.87	1,417.98	3,066.83	3,340.49	2,909.93
Self-employment	1,324.34	1,160.33	516.41	245.60	392.65
Dividends and interest	746.60	915.18	1,389.82	879.83	991.75
Rents	189.35	273.70	222.32	194.25	213.44
Unemployment	98.26	74.35	64.68	45.49	24.79
Welfare, public assistance	71.43	87.21	74.57	85.66	136.75
Other sources	231.56	188.67	122.77	66.95	62.22
Total income	$14,232.61	$11,555.96	$8,141.71	$6,262.83	$5,339.97

Source: Consumer Expenditure Survey, 1972–73.

welfare and public assistance, including old-age assistance, aid to families with dependent children, disability insurance, and food stamp benefits. The decreasing importance of earnings and the increasing importance of retirement benefits with increasing age of the household head was evident in each year. Increases in some of the other sources of income were not sufficient to offset the decreased earnings, causing the decline in total income with age.

These groupings of income sources differ slightly from published tabulations by the Bureau of Labor Statistics. For example, food stamp benefits were included as one of the components of "other sources" in our analysis rather than in the welfare and public assistance category. In addition, we included the net profit from the purchase and sales of stocks and bonds within the same calendar year with dividends and interest. We also included income from subleasing with income from rental property and workmen's compensation with unemployment income.

Differences in per capita income were not as great as the variation in total income with age because of decreasing household size, with the oldest group containing approximately one less person on the average than the youngest group. Nevertheless, total income decreased faster than household size, resulting in a decrease in per capita income.

Self-employment income did not decline with age as soon as other earnings, but the change was fairly distinct for the groups aged 65 and older relative to the two younger groups. There was a tendency for the importance of dividends, interest, and rents to increase with age, but the relationships were not the same between 1972 and 1973. The amount of income received from government transfers other than social security and other sources was insignificant for all age groups, never exceeding 3.8 percent of total income. In comparing these results with those from the RHS and the PSID reported earlier, it is important to remember that here separate groups of individuals of the same age were compared over time. In contrast, the RHS and PSID data showed changes in the same cohort over time as the couples aged.

Income Differences by Race

When the set of elderly households was classified by race, a much smaller increase in total income was observed for black households than for nonblack households between 1972 and 1973. Average income for nonblacks in 1973 was nearly 15.2 percent higher than comparable values for 1972, whereas the comparable value for blacks was only 3 percent higher than the previous year. In per capita terms, income of blacks was actually less in 1973 than in 1972, because differences in average family size in the samples for the two years more than offset the differences in total incomes. The average household size for the black group in 1973 was 2.29 persons, compared to 2.08 in 1972.

One reason for the large differences in annual changes for the two races was that between 1972 and 1973 earnings and self-employment income decreased for blacks but increased for nonblacks. Retirement benefits and other sources of income increased for both races between 1972 and 1973. Returns from capital assets were not very large in either year for blacks relative to nonblacks. Differences in capital assets along with earnings and self-employment income explain why total income for blacks averaged only slightly over 50 percent of nonblack total income. Many of the same patterns observed in Table 4.9 were also noted when the observations for the nonblack households were classified by age. This is not surprising since the nonblack group comprised more than 90 percent of the total sample each year. The racial categories in this discussion (black/nonblack) differ from those used in describing the RHS data (white/nonwhite). These categories are not identical and are used because of the reporting in the two surveys.

Marital Status

The substantial year-to-year differences in total incomes for married and single females were also observed. Generally, year-to-year differences were greatest among married households for the under-65 age groups, whereas they were largest among single females in the 65–74 age group. The 55–64 married household groups had substantial increases in earnings, self-employment income, and dividends and interest, as well as retirement benefits between 1972 and 1973. Most of the year-to-year differences for single females between the ages of 65 and 69 occurred in dividends and interest as well as in retirement benefits. The latter categories as well as earnings were responsible for the 34.2 percent difference in total income for the 70–74 age group. The large difference in earnings for the latter group may reflect sample variability more than year-to-year changes.

Many other relationships, such as the declining importance of earnings and increasing dependence on retirement benefits with age, were quite similar for single females and married households. Overall, however, married households were a little less dependent on retirement benefits and derived more of their income from earnings and self-employment than single females of similar age.

REVIEW OF OTHER EMPIRICAL RESEARCH ON INCOMES OF THE ELDERLY COHORTS

Several other studies that have recently examined the trend of the real income of the elderly cohorts provide general support for the findings of this study.

Using the March Current Population Surveys (CPS), Bridges and Packard (1981) examined the 1970 elderly cohort consisting of persons who were 65 and older in 1970. By following persons of similar age (66 and over in 1971, 67 and over in 1972, etc.) in successive years, the trend in income of an elderly cohort can be approximated. This analysis is similar to our cohort analysis, but it differs in that the same individuals are not followed over time. Instead, a hypothetical cohort is formed by following in future surveys different people who were born in the same years. Table 4.10 shows that the real income of this constructed cohort rose slightly between 1970 and 1974 but declined by 5.6 percent from 1974 to 1977. As expected, real earnings dropped sharply as the cohort aged. This was primarily in response to a decline from 41 percent in 1970 to 23 percent in 1977 in the proportion of families with earnings.

The rise in real income between 1970 and 1974 is attributable to the large increase in social security benefits. During the eight years, the proportion of the cohort receiving benefits rose by 12 percent, and average real benefits per recipient family increased by 30 percent. The legislated and automatic increases totaled 33 percent. The greater real increase of social security in the first part of the period was due to higher retirement rates among families aged 65 to 69 (thereby increasing the number of recipients) and the shift from legislated to automatic increases in social security benefits.

Hurd and Shoven (1982b) examined the RHS data and found that real income of the couples fell by approximately 10 percent between 1968 and 1974. This decline is smaller than that reported earlier in this chapter because Hurd and Shoven included the imputed value of home ownership, medicare,

TABLE 4.10. Average Real Income of Persons 65 and Older in 1970, 1970–77

Source	Real Income			Percent of Total		
	1970	1974	1977	1970	1974	1977
Earnings	$1,795	$1,160	$ 830	40	25	19
Property income	750	855	900	17	19	21
Social security benefits	1,265	1,800	1,840	28	39	43
Other transfer income	685	745	735	15	16	17
Total	$4,495	$4,565	$4,305	100	100	100

Source: Benjamin Bridges and Michael Packard. "Price and Income Changes for the Elderly," *Social Security Bulletin* 44 (January 1981): 10.
Note: Values in 1967 dollars.

and medicaid. The real income of some groups of the single men and women actually rose during the period.

Hurd and Shoven (1982b) also analyzed the wealth of the RHS cohort. They found that the total wealth of these persons increased between 1969 and 1975. Their measure of wealth included pensions, social security, medicare, home, and other financial assets. In addition, they examined the vulnerability of wealth to loss in real value with inflation. Their findings suggested only small declines in the real wealth of the RHS cohort with price increases, and this decline was concentrated among wealthier individuals.

Barnes and Zedlewski (1981) also examined the RHS for changes in real income. They reported life-cycle patterns of income declines that were generally consistent with those in our study. For most of their subgroups, real income rose during retirement. They found that real income from pensions and financial assets declined for retirees. The real income of full-time workers continued to rise except for the oldest of the respondents.

RISING REAL INCOME OF PERSONS AGED 65 AND OVER

Most of the discussion in this chapter has been based on cohort analysis, which examined changes in the income of a group of individuals as they aged. An alternative method of examining trends in real income of older persons is to follow the income of a specific age group over time. This income series holds age constant but includes cohort effects as new people enter the group through aging and others exit from the group. Data of this kind are frequently used in debates on the well-being of the elderly. In the following analysis, the median real cash income of the elderly is used to indicate the trend in income of persons 65 and over. To a large extent this method enables us to examine trends in income of older persons holding constant the important event of retirement.

The median income, deflated by the CPI, of families whose head is aged 65 or older rose by almost 100 percent between 1950 and 1980. This rising real

TABLE 4.11. Real Median Family Income, 1950–82

Year	Head of Family 65 and Over[a] (1)	Head of Family Aged 45–54[a] (2)	Relative Income of Elderly Families $(1 \div 2) \times 100$
1950	$2,639	$ 5,110	51.6
1955	2,900	6,344	45.7
1960	3,266	7,303	44.7
1961	3,377	7,491	45.1
1962	3,536	7,770	45.5
1963	3,655	8,086	45.2
1964	3,634	8,344	43.6
1965	3,661	8,717	42.0
1966	3,750	9,116	41.1
1967	3,927	9,676	40.6
1968	4,348	10,012	43.4
1969	4,374	10,561	41.4
1970	4,345	10,422	41.7
1971	4,495	10,706	42.0
1972	4,763	11,218	42.5
1973	4,827	11,437	42.2
1974	5,081	11,210	45.3
1975	4,998	10,899	45.9
1976	5,115	11,165	45.8
1977	5,019	11,478	43.7
1978	5,193	11,580	44.8
1979	5,202	11,661	44.6
1980	5,215	11,035	47.3
1981	5,264	10,733	49.1
1982	5,575	10,629	52.5

Source: U.S. Bureau of the Census, *Current Population Reports,* Series P-60, various years.

[a] Values derived by deflating nominal income by CPI (1967 = 100).

income of the elderly is shown in Table 4.11. Compared to that of all families, the relative income of older families declined by 10 percent in the 1950s, remained fairly stable during the 1960s, and rose by 20 percent during the 1970s. Because the median income of all families can be substantially affected by the age composition of the population, real income of older families is compared in Table 4.11 to the income of families whose head is aged 45 to 54. Heads of the latter familes are in their peak earnings years, so the ratio of the income of elderly families to that of families with heads aged 45 to 54 years will be lower than the ratio of their relative income compared to that of all families. When compared to that of middle-aged families, the relative income of older families fell by 13.4 percent during the 1950s and by 6.7 percent in the 1960s, before rising by 13.4 percent during the 1970s (see Table 4.12). During these decades, the consumer price index rose by 23.3 percent, 31.1 percent, and 112.4 percent respectively. Thus the loss in relative income for elderly families was greatest when inflation was lowest, and there was a

TABLE 4.12. Change in Real and Relative Income, 1950–80

	Percentage Increase in Real Cash Median Income		Percentage Change in Relative Income of Elderly[a]	Percentage Change in Consumer Price Index
Period	Family Head Aged 65 and Over	Family Head Aged 45 to 54		
1950–60	23.8	42.9	– 13.4	23.3
1960–70	33.0	42.7	– 6.7	31.1
1970–80	20.0	5.9	13.4	112.4

Source: Columns 1, 2, and 3 are derived from information in Table 4.11. Column 4 is derived from CPI data shown in Council of Economic Advisers, *Economic Report of the President* (Washington, D.C.: Government Printing Office, 1983), Table B-52, p. 221.

[a] Percentage change from last column of Table 4.11.

significant gain in relative income during the high inflation decade of the 1970s. The rise in relative income of the elderly may have occurred because of the virtual cessation of real economic growth during the 1970s, which stopped the growth in the real income of workers. By contrast, the real income of the elderly continued to rise with increases in the real value of government transfers.

The improving relative income position of the elderly was also indicated in research by Danziger et al. (1982), Hurd and Shoven (1982a), and Bridges and Packard (1981). Danziger et al. show that the median income of families whose head was aged 65 and over rose steadily from 49 percent of the median income of all families in 1966 to 64 percent in 1981. Thus, the relative income of the elderly in comparison with the general population rose by almost one-third in fifteen years. Hurd and Shoven included in their measure of income the imputed returns from home ownership and the cash value of medicare and medicaid benefits. Using this broader measure of income, the ratio of income per elderly household to income of the entire population rose from 52 percent in 1970 to 58 percent in 1978.

Bridges and Packard examined trends in mean real income of persons 65 and over. They found that the average real income of families whose head was 65 and older rose by approximately 10 percent between 1970 and 1977, while the average real income of the nonelderly families was approximately constant during the same period. The average real income of the elderly rose as a percent of the income of the nonelderly from 49 to 54 percent between 1970 and 1977, with all this improvement occurring between 1970 and 1974. In their study the nominal income of the elderly was deflated by an older person CPI, whereas the income of the nonelderly was deflated using the CPI for workers (see Chapter 3 for a description of these indexes developed by Bridges and Packard).

A final indicator in the improving economic status of the elderly is the decline in the incidence of poverty for older Americans. Table 4.13 shows the

TABLE 4.13. Poverty Rates of the Elderly and Total Population, 1959–82

	Elderly		Total Population	
Year	Poverty Rate	Number of Persons (in millions)	Poverty Rate	Number of Persons (in millions)
1959	32.2	5.5	22.4	39.5
1968	25.0	4.6	12.8	25.4
1969	25.3	4.8	12.1	24.1
1970	24.5	4.7	12.6	25.4
1971	21.6	4.3	12.5	25.6
1972	18.6	3.7	11.9	24.5
1973	16.3	3.4	11.1	23.0
1974	15.7	3.3	11.6	24.3
1975	15.3	3.3	12.3	25.9
1976	15.0	3.3	11.8	25.0
1977	14.1	3.2	11.6	24.7
1978	14.0	3.2	11.4	24.5
1979	15.2	3.7	11.6	25.3
1980	15.7	3.9	13.0	29.3
1981	15.3	3.9	14.0	31.8
1982	14.6	3.8	15.0	34.4

Source: U.S. Bureau of the Census, *Current Population Reports,* Series P-60, no. 127, "Money Income and Poverty Status of Families and Persons in the United States: 1980" (Advance Data from the March 1981 Current Population Survey) (Washington, D.C.: Government Printing Office, 1981), p. 29; and U.S. Bureau of the Census, *Current Population Reports,* Series P-60, no. 140, "Money Income and Poverty Status of Families and Persons in the United States: 1982" (Washington, D.C.: Government Printing Office, 1983), p. 4.

trend in the poverty rate for the elderly and for the total population in selected years during the past two decades. The poverty rate for persons aged 65 and older declined from 24.5 percent in 1970 to 14.6 percent in 1982. By contrast, the poverty rate for all persons declined slightly between 1970 and 1978 before rising by almost four percentage points to 15 percent in 1982, when for the first time the poverty rate for the elderly was below the national rate. Danziger et al. (1982) showed that the rate of decline in the incidence of poverty of all white older families exceeded the decline for black- and female-headed older households.

These aggregate age-group data indicate that the relative income of persons 65 and over improved significantly during the high-inflation decade of the 1970s. This improvement has continued during the first years of the 1980s as the rate of inflation has declined.

In this chapter we looked at a series of longitudinal surveys and other national data to determine the effect of inflation on the real income of the elderly. On the basis of this analysis, we can conclude that the elderly were not more adversely affected by inflation than were other demographic groups. Life-cycle income patterns of declining income at retirement continue to exist, but there is no evidence that inflation significantly altered this decline. The 1970s was a period of relatively high rates of inflation, and during that time the real and relative incomes of older Americans rose. Of course, some groups of older persons were more protected from inflation than others. For example, the real income of low-income persons grew more rapidly than the income of higher-income elderly. In the next two chapters we will look at specific income sources and suggest why incomes of certain groups of older persons were more responsive to changes in prices.

5 Federal Transfer Programs to the Elderly

During the past half-century, the federal government has played an increasing role in determining the economic well-being of the elderly. The growth and development of cash and in-kind benefit programs has significantly altered the sources of income for most older persons and changed their vulnerability to unanticipated price changes. Federal expenditures on the elderly include payments through retirement programs, old-age, survivors, and disability insurance (OASDI), health-care subsidies, welfare programs, housing assistance, and social services. Table 5.1 lists the specific programs and the costs of old-age transfers from these programs in fiscal year 1982. Total federal expenditures on these programs for individuals aged 65 and over were $196.2 billion (U.S. Congressional Budget Office, 1982; see also Califano, 1978).

The long-term improvement in the real income of the elderly, described in Chapter 4, has been accelerated by the expansion in coverage and the increase of benefits of social security and other income maintenance programs, as well as by the initiation of additional income transfer programs. In this chapter we

TABLE 5.1. Estimated Federal Outlays for Persons 65 and Older, by Program, Fiscal Year 1982 (in Billions of Dollars)

Program	Outlays
Social security	111.8
Medicare	39.7
Other federal retirement and survivor programs	21.1
Medicaid	6.5
Veterans benefits	4.3
Housing assistance	3.3
Supplemental security income	2.9
Other federal health programs	2.3
Administration on aging	0.7
Food stamps	0.6
Title XX social services	0.4
Energy assistance	0.2
Other	2.4
Total	196.2

Source: U.S. Congressional Budget Office, *Work and Retirement: Options for Continued Employment of Older Workers* (Washington, D.C.: Government Printing Office, July 1982), p. 55.

will see how the increased importance of transfer payments has altered the vulnerability of the elderly to losses in real income due to inflation.

GROWTH IN FEDERAL SPENDING

Federal expenditures on behalf of persons aged 65 and over have risen dramatically since the early 1960s in response to legislative initiatives and growth in the older population. Benefit programs for the elderly are estimated to have totaled $12.8 billion in 1960, whereas expenditures in 1982 reached $196.2 billion, a fifteen-fold increase (see Table 5.2). By contrast, the number of people aged 65 and over increased by only 57.5 percent over the same period — from 16.7 million in 1960 to 26.3 million in July 1981. These expenditure figures do not include the value of preferential tax treatment given the elderly.

Between 1960 and 1982 the consumer price index more than tripled. As a result, federal expenditures for the elderly measured in 1967 dollars were $14.4 billion in 1960, and real spending on these programs in 1982 was five times the 1960 level. Thus, two-thirds of the growth in annual spending on the elderly can be attributed to price increases, but still there has been a significant increase in the real resources allocated to these programs. Reflecting this real increase is the growth in the proportion of the federal budget necessary to finance these programs from 13 percent in 1960 to 27 percent in 1982. A similar increase is noted in the proportion of the gross national product allocated to these benefit programs, from 2.5 percent to 5.9 percent (see Califano, 1978; Torrey, 1982).

The average annual benefit per person aged 65 and over increased from $768 in 1960 to $7,948 in 1982 (see Table 5.3). If benefits had been increased

TABLE 5.2. Annual Federal Expenditures for Persons Aged 65 and Older, 1960–82

Year	Total Expenditures (Billions)	Total Expenditures in 1967 Dollars[a] (Billions)	Percentage of GNP	Percentage of Federal Budget
1960	$ 12.8	$14.4	2.5	13
1965	18.8	19.9	2.7	16
1970	38.2	32.8	3.9	19
1975	75.7	47.0	4.9	23
1978	112.5	57.6	5.3	24
1982	196.2	67.9	5.9	27

Source: Robert Clark and John Menefee, "Federal Expenditures for the Elderly," *The Gerontologist* 21 (April 1981): 132–37. The 1982 figures are based on estimates from U.S. Congressional Budget Office, *Work and Retirement* (Washington, D.C.: Government Printing Office, July 1982); and Barbara Torrey, "Guns vs. Canes: The Fiscal Implications of an Aging Population," *American Economic Review* 72 (May 1982): 309–13. The 1982 data pertain to fiscal year 1982.

[a] Nominal dollar values are deflated by annual averages of monthly figures of the CPI.

TABLE 5.3. Annual Federal Expenditures per Person Aged 65 and Older, 1960–82

Year	Actual Expenditures	Benefits Rise to Reflect Price Increases	Benefits Rise to Reflect Growth in Per Capita Disposable Income
1960	$ 768	$ 768	$ 768
1965	1,019	818	966
1970	1,902	1,007	1,337
1975	3,379	1,396	2,002
1978	4,678	1,692	2,592
1982	7,948	2,516	3,663

Source: Table 5.2 and U.S. population and economic data. The price increases are determined using the CPI.

only to reflect price increases, the average benefit would have been $2,516 in 1982, but if benefits had risen in accordance with the growth in per capita disposable income, the transfer per elderly person would have been $3,663. Therefore, the expansion in federal spending per older American since 1960 has significantly exceeded the growth of annual per capita income. This increase is the result of the introduction of new programs, higher benefits under existing programs, and less restrictive eligibility conditions.

The relevant data reveal that the increase in the numbers of aged has been a significant factor in the rise in aggregate spending on the nation's elderly. But expenditures have not been driven up uncontrollably by a graying of the population; instead, most of the increase is due to the federal government's response to the perceived needs and/or the growing political power of the elderly with improvements in the income maintenance system.

New programs have been introduced, and benefits under existing programs have been liberalized and coverage expanded. Thus, much of the past graying of the federal budget has occurred because of explicit policy changes by the federal government (Clark and Menefee, 1981). One important change in federal policy has been the indexing of government programs to changes in consumer prices. Indexing provisions reduce the lag time of increases in benefits from ad hoc adjustments. Specific programs are examined below for their responsiveness to increases in consumer prices.

INDEXING OF FEDERAL INCOME TRANSFER PROGRAMS

The levels and rates of change of benefits to older persons are determined by congressional action. Most of the rapid growth in benefits outlined above has been because of specific legislation increasing benefits, expanding coverage, and/or instituting new programs. One of the most important innovations has been the indexing of benefit programs to changes in the cost of living. The Federal Civil Service Retirement System was the first major program for which automatic pension benefit increases were tied to increases in the consumer price index. This legislation, enacted in 1962, was followed the next year by the indexing of pension benefits for military retirees. The first indexing of income-tested programs occurred in 1971, when Congress required that food stamp allotments automatically rise each year with food prices. Presently, eighty-six federal programs now have one or more provisions that increase in response to a rise in some index, usually a measure of prices or wages (U.S. Congressional Research Service, 1981). The programs most important to the income of the elderly are reviewed below.

Old Age and Survivors Insurance

The initial U.S. social security legislation was passed in 1935, considerably later than most other industrialized countries. At first, only retired workers aged 65 and older were eligible for benefits. In 1939, benefits were extended to dependents with the initiation of a 50 percent spouse benefit and a benefit for widows. Subsequent amendments permitted workers to retire between the ages of 62 and 65 at reduced benefits, and incorporated disability benefits into this system of income protection.

Initially, workers in commerce and industry (except railroads) under the age of 65 in the United States were mandatorily covered by social security. Subsequent expansions in coverage have added farm and domestic workers, farmers, and other self-employed workers. These extensions have raised social security coverage from 58 percent of the paid labor force in 1940 to approximately 90 percent in 1982. Legislation enacted in 1983 extended coverage to include all federal workers hired after January 1, 1984, and employees of nonprofit organizations. In addition, state and local governmental units will not be permitted to withdraw from coverage in the future. Thus, the future coverage rate should increase to approximately 100 percent.

Social security benefits are determined by applying a specified formula to a person's earnings history. If the recipient has other sources of income, his or her right to receive benefits is unimpaired as long as the recipient is not currently working for the income. The basic benefit for those who retire at age 65 is determined by a benefit formula that replaces a portion of the average indexed monthly earnings (AIME) of the recipient. The replacement rate falls as the AIME rises. Benefits are reduced for early retirement between the ages of 62 and 65 and increased for delayed retirement after age 65. Additional benefits are provided for dependents and widows.

Prior to 1972, individual benefit payments were raised by specific legislative amendments enacted every few years. An automatic adjustment for changes in the cost of living was adopted in 1972. The ad hoc benefit increases and the post-1972 automatic increases have been sufficient to raise the real level of benefits since the early 1960s. The cumulative effect of statutory and automatic increases in primary insurance benefits under OASDI was a minimum increase in the primary insurance benefit of 210 percent between

January 1965 and June 1980, compared to a 160 percent change in the consumer price index. Subsequent automatic increases have been sufficient to maintain the real value of benefits during the 1980s. These increases, along with a growth in real earnings, have raised the average monthly benefit of retired workers from $22 in 1940 to over $420 for those receiving benefits in 1983, when over 25 million persons aged 65 and over were receiving benefits. These increases were sufficient to raise the benefit to preretirement earnings ratio for single middle-income workers from approximately 30 percent in the late 1960s to almost 45 percent by the middle 1970s (see Munnell, 1977, p. 64; Rosen, 1981; Fox, 1979). This ratio is often referred to as a replacement rate and measures the proportion of earnings just prior to retirement replaced by social security benefits.

Much of this increase in the replacement ratio after 1972 was an unintended side effect of the automatic adjustment mechanism instituted in 1972. The method of adjustment of benefits with respect to inflation worked as expected for persons already retired but overcompensated future retirees. As a result, the replacement rate for new retirees rose with increases in inflation (Campbell, 1976; Kaplan, 1977). Legislation in 1977 removed this overcompensation effect. As examined below, the new law indexed past wages in a manner that provides for a constant replacement ratio in the future.

Total OASDI expenditures have risen because of the introduction of new programs, expansion of coverage, and increases in the level of benefits. Payments have also increased with the maturing of the system as more people have become eligible based on their work histories. These factors have generated an income security program that has required an increasing proportion of national income to finance its benefit payments. Total benefits paid have risen from $1 million in 1937 to $961 million in 1950, $18 billion in 1965, and an estimated $170 billion in 1983. As a result, this program, which required less than one-tenth of a percent of the nation's personal income in the early 1940s and only 2.8 percent in 1960, now requires approximately 7 percent of personal income to meet current expenditures. Table 5.4 shows the significant rise in the payroll tax required to finance the OASDI program as it has matured, been liberalized, and felt the effect of population aging. The 1983 legislation rescheduled a series of tax increases throughout the 1980s and provides for an ultimate tax rate for OASDI of 6.20 percent of payroll to be paid by the employee and an equal rate paid by the employer.

As noted above, a number of the provisions of benefit determination of the old age, survivors, and disability insurance (OASDI) program are indexed to either wages or prices. Postretirement benefits are indexed to the CPI for urban wage and clerical workers and are increased annually in January if this index has risen by 3 percent or more during the period from the third quarter of one year to the corresponding quarter of the next. A declining CPI would not lower benefits. This adjustment mechanism was established in 1972 and

TABLE 5.4. Annual Maximum Taxable Earnings and Actual Contribution Rates: Old Age, Survivors, Disability, and Health Insurance

Beginning	Annual Maximum Taxable Earnings	Tax Rate (Percent)			
		Total	Employer and Employee, Each		
			OASI	DI	HI
1937	$ 3,000	1.000	1.000	–	–
1950	3,000	1.500	1.500	–	–
1951	3,600	1.500	1.500	–	–
1954	3,600	2.000	2.000	–	–
1955	4,200	2.000	2.000	–	–
1957	4,200	2.250	2.000	0.25	–
1959	4,800	2.500	2.250	0.25	–
1960	4,800	3.000	2.750	0.25	–
1962	4,800	3.125	2.875	0.25	–
1963	4,800	3.625	3.375	0.25	–
1966	6,600	4.200	3.500	0.35	0.35
1967	6,600	4.400	3.550	0.35	0.50
1968	7,800	4.400	3.325	0.475	0.60
1969	7,800	4.800	3.725	0.475	0.60
1970	7,800	4.800	3.650	0.55	0.60
1971	7,800	5.200	4.050	0.55	0.60
1972	9,000	5.200	4.050	0.55	0.60
1973	10,800	5.850	4.300	0.55	1.00
1974	13,200	5.850	4.375	0.575	0.90
1975	14,100	5.850	4.375	0.575	0.90
1976	15,300	5.850	4.375	0.575	0.90
1977	16,500	5.850	4.375	0.575	0.90
1978	17,700	6.050	4.275	0.775	1.00
1979	22,900	6.130	4.330	0.75	1.05
1980	25,900	6.130	4.330	0.75	1.05
1981	29,700	6.650	4.525	0.825	1.30
1982	32,400	6.700	4.575	0.825	1.30
1983	35,700	6.700	4.775	0.625	1.30

Source: U.S. Social Security Administration, *Social Security Bulletin: Annual Statistical Supplement, 1977–79,* p. 35; and *1982 Annual Report of the Board of Trustees of the Federal Old Age and Survivors Insurance and Disability Insurance Trust Funds.*

amended in 1977 to prevent early retirees from receiving benefit increases in excess of the CPI increase. Initially, benefit increases were awarded in July, but the 1983 social security amendments delayed the cost-of-living adjustment for 1983 until January 1984 and established January of each year as the time for future increases. These amendments also limited future increases to the lesser of the increases in wages or prices if the ratio of the combined OASDI trust fund assets to estimated expenditures falls below a specified percentage. The ratio that institutes this limitation is 15 percent through December 1988 and 20 percent thereafter.

The earnings test reduces benefits by $1 for every $2 a beneficiary earns in excess of a specified exempt amount – $6,600 for those between the ages of 65 and 69 in 1983. After 1982, exempt earnings have been adjusted annually, effective January 1, by the rise in average wages. The exempted amount for retirees aged 62 to 65 was indexed starting in 1979. The raising of the earnings limit with average wages means that the real earnings of beneficiaries will not be reduced as inflation raises their nominal earnings for the same number of hours of work.

Initial social security benefits are also indexed to average wage growth. When individuals first become eligible for benefits, their average indexed monthly wage (AIME) is calculated by indexing past earnings by the rate of wage growth between 1951 and the year of eligibility. The AIME is then used to determine the primary insurance amount by a progressive benefit formula. For a person born in 1917 who first became eligible for benefits at age 62 in 1979, the 1983 formula was 90 percent of the first $180 of the AIME plus 32 percent of the amount above $180 up to $1,085, plus 15 percent of any amount in excess of $1,085. These dollar amounts or bend points in the formula are indexed to the rate of increase in average wages so that persons born after 1917 have higher bend points. This indexing maintains a constant replacement ratio over time for OASDI beneficiaries; that is, benefits for future retirees are rising at a rate equal to the growth of wages.

The taxable earnings base is indexed to increases in the average wage in the economy. Also indexed to average wages are the family maximum benefit and the earnings level required for one quarter of coverage. The special minimum benefit is indexed to the CPI and adjusted annually.

Social security benefits are a significant source of income to millions of older Americans. In 1983, some 25 million persons aged 65 and older received retired workers or survivor and dependent benefits. Thus, the indexing of social security benefits (and before that, the ad hoc congressional increases) means that the dominant source of income for older persons is basically unaffected by inflation.

Federal Pensions

Pension benefits for federal government employees began with the payment of benefits to soldiers who fought in the Revolutionary War. The Federal Civil Service Retirement System was established in 1920 and expanded by amendments in 1942 and 1946 to include employees in the executive, judicial, and legislative branches of the government. Separate retirement systems have been developed for other federal employees. Over time these programs have been expanded and liberalized to provide increased benefits for retirees (Greenough and King, 1976). Increased funding has also been necessary because of the expanded size of the federal government labor force that with a lag increases the number of beneficiaries. The cost of federal pensions has gone up because of full (and at times over) indexation of benefits for increases in consumer prices. Expenditures for the civil service retirement system were estimated to be $17.6 billion in fiscal year 1981, up from $15 billion in fiscal 1980.

The federal government has different retirement programs for alternative groups of workers. These systems include the federal civil service, military, foreign service, Federal Reserve Board employees, comptrollers general, and Central Intelligence Agency retirement systems. Benefits were first indexed in 1962, and until recently retirement benefits in these programs have been increased to reflect fully changes in the CPI. Legislation in the summer of 1982 delayed the inflation adjustment by one month in each of the next three years. In addition, retirees who have not reached age 62 will receive an increase of only 50 percent of the change in the CPI.

Supplemental Security Income

Supplemental security income (SSI), which was instituted in 1974 to replace the old-age assistance program, guarantees a minimum monthly level of income to the aged. It is a welfare program financed from general tax revenues. Unlike social security, a history of work in covered employment is irrelevant in determining eligibility and the level of benefits. Instead, eligibility is determined by certain income and assets tests. The SSI program reduces benefits dollar for dollar for unearned income above $20 a month and 50 cents for every $1 of monthly earned income above $65. The effect of these tests is that SSI directs income to the poorest of the elderly much more accurately than does social security. Despite this target population, there is a relatively low participation rate in this program. Menefee et al. (1981) estimate that only 55 percent of the eligible low-income elderly population is enrolled in SSI.

In July 1982 some 1.6 million elderly persons received federally administered SSI benefits averaging $154 a month. Table 5.5 indicates that the number of people receiving these benefits has declined since 1974, but the average

TABLE 5.5. Supplemental Security Income: Federally Administered Payments, 1974–82

Year[a]	Number of Aged Beneficiaries (Millions)	Average Monthly Benefits
1974	2.3	$ 91.60
1975	2.3	90.93
1976	2.1	94.37
1977	2.1	96.62
1978	2.0	100.43
1979	1.9	122.67
1980	1.8	128.20
1981	1.7	136.06
1982	1.6	154.13

Source: Lenna Kennedy, "SSI Trends and Changes, 1974–1980," *Social Security Bulletin,* July 1982, pp. 3–12, and *Social Security Bulletin,* November 1982, p. 48.
[a] All values are for December of designated year except 1982 data, which are for July.

benefit has risen slightly in nominal terms. State-administered state supplementary SSI programs have an additional 130,000 beneficiaries.

SSI benefits are increased annually when the CPI has increased by more than 3 percent during the preceding year. States are no longer allowed to reduce their supplement when the federal government raises its payments. Other components of the system (e.g., income standards, income disregards, and allowable asset levels) are not indexed.

GOVERNMENT IN-KIND TRANSFERS AND THE WELL-BEING OF THE ELDERLY

In addition to cash payments, the government provides older persons benefits in the form of specific goods and services. Most of these benefits are in the form of food, housing, and health care. Some programs transfer the commodity directly to the elderly, while other programs allow older persons to consume the good at reduced prices. The largest of these programs is medicare, which provides medical insurance to virtually all persons over age 65. Most of the other in-kind benefit programs are poverty programs that provide benefits to low-income families.

It is difficult to determine the effect of in-kind benefit programs on the well-being of individuals. Clearly, if a person elects to participate in a voluntary in-kind benefit program, his or her well-being is improved. The model developed in Chapters 1 and 2 can be used to show this. However, the magnitude of this improvement is less obvious. When a cash transfer is received, the individual's ability to consume all goods and services is increased, and the individual can select the set of commodities to maximize well-being. In contrast, the recipient of a specific commodity through an in-kind benefit program is required to consume all these new resources in the form of that commodity. Unless the recipient can sell or trade the commodity in a secondary market, no substitution across goods can be achieved. As a result, money transfers will always improve family well-being by more than an in-kind benefit of equal cash value.

The appropriate method of evaluating in-kind benefits has been examined by Moon (1977, 1979), Smeeding (1982), Paglin (1980), Borzilleri (1980), and Moon and Smolensky (1977). Some of this research attempts to measure the gain in well-being from in-kind benefits in relation to a cash transfer, but such an extension is beyond the scope of this research. Instead, the cost to the government of providing the in-kind transfer to older persons is derived, and it is assumed that this would be the cost to the individual of acquiring this commodity in the marketplace. This value is then considered as the gain in family resources from participating in the program. This method will in most cases overstate the true improvement in the well-being of the recipients. This overvaluing of the in-kind benefit is especially important when family income is being compared with a cash value poverty level (Moon, 1979).

Federal Health Policy

The role of the federal government in health policy began in the late 1800s with issues involving public health measures. In the early 1900s, the impetus shifted toward the government's responsibility for the health of the individual. Theodore Roosevelt made national health insurance an issue in his campaign for the presidency in 1912, but movement toward a comprehensive health policy has been slow (Feder et al., 1980). It was not until 1950 that federal participation in payments for medical care became possible in most public assistance programs. The social security amendments of that year allowed federal public assistance categorical grants-in-aid to include federal cost-sharing in charges for hospital and medical care paid by state welfare agencies. Payments were limited to persons on the welfare rolls. Support for the health needs of the elderly was not directly provided until 1960 with enactment of the 1960 Social Security Amendments, the Kerr-Mills Act, which authorized matching grants to states for medical assistance for the aged. This open-ended federal cost-sharing program had no limitations on payments to individuals or on total state expenditures. State participation was optional and the states were given the responsibility for cost control. However, coverage was severely limited by the program's stringent eligibility rules, variability in state participation, and the costs to the states. Even the lure of high rates of federal matching funds was not sufficient to entice some states to establish medical assistance programs (Stevens and Stevens, 1974).

In 1965 medicare was enacted, replacing the Kerr-Mills approach by a uniform, compulsory hospital insurance program (HI) financed by a payroll tax and a supplementary medical insurance plan (SMI) financed through direct payment and federal subsidies. Amended in 1967 and 1972 to clarify services and eligibility as well as to try to contain costs and achieve administrative control, the medicare approach has taken much of the health care of the elderly out of the welfare system (see Myers, chaps. 7–9). Under HI, the elderly receive reimbursement or subsidization for in-patient hospital services, extended care, and posthospitalization home visits. The supplemental insurance of SMI allows subsidized physician services, diagnostic tests, and some other nonhospital services. Individuals must still pay deductible amounts and pay for uncovered services. Low-income elderly are eligible for additional medical assistance through medicaid, which was also instituted by legislation in 1965. For those eligible for low-income assistance, this program can pay for charges not covered by medicare.

Total disbursements under the hospital insurance program have risen from $3.4 billion in 1967 to an estimated $41 billion in 1983. The corresponding payroll tax rates for HI are shown in Table 5.4. Government contributions to the supplementary medical insurance plan have increased from $667 million in 1967 to an estimated $14 billion in 1983. These cost figures were driven up by medical-care cost increases that were more than twice that which could be attributed to general wage and price increases. Part of the cost increase is due to the greater use of health services, implying an increase in the average health care of the elderly. Factors increasing payments through the health insurance programs have also stimulated higher medicaid payments. Medical assistance benefits to the aged through medicaid were $6.5 billion in fiscal year 1982. Medical expenditures have been rising so rapidly that these programs threaten to become a major fiscal concern in the coming decades (Torrey, 1982; O'Neill, 1978). Legislation during the early 1980s has attempted to slow the growth in costs by reducing benefits and raising fees for SMI.

Since medicare is the largest government program providing in-kind benefits to older persons, it is important that the value of these benefits be included in an assessment of the well-being of the elderly. Two significant conceptual issues arise in the evaluation of these benefits. First, should the value of medical services actually received be a measure of medicare benefits? If utilization of the program is the measure of benefits, then people who are in poorer health and therefore consume more health services will be viewed as having more resources and higher well-being than persons with better health. To avoid this result, an insurance value of health benefits is derived. The second issue pertains to an individual's evaluation of the health insurance. If a person would not purchase this quantity of insurance at current market prices if given an equal amount of cash, then the cash value of the health insurance overstates the actual value to the individual. This possibility is not directly addressed. Chapters 1 and 2 contain a theoretical discussion of some of these issues.

The insurance value for the two parts of medicare is determined by adding annual health care payments and administrative costs and then dividing this sum by the number of enrollees. All enrollee contributions are then deducted to determine the net value of medical insurance. Several assumptions are implicit in this derivation of an insurance value of the health insurance program. If the benefit is to be compared with the insurance a person would purchase in the market without a government medical assistance program, then it must be assumed that this program has not altered medical prices and that the administrative cost does not differ from that in the private sector. It could be argued that a normal profit rate should be included in the value of insurance because private producers of this service would require a return on investment. The exclusion of this term implies that the insurance is evaluated at the actual cost to the government and not at the fair market price an individual would face in the private economy (Smeeding, 1982).

The value of uniform health insurance will vary across individuals on the basis of their current health and the availability of medical facilities and the

TABLE 5.6. Health Insurance: Number of Beneficiaries and Level of Benefits, 1966–81

Year	No. of Enrollees[a] (Thousands)	Disbursements (Millions)			Nominal Insurance Value[b]	Real Insurance Value[c]
		Benefits	Administrative Expenditures	Total Disbursements		
1966	19,082	$ 891	$108	$ 999	$ 52.35	$ 53.86
1967	19,494	3,353	77	3,430	175.95	175.95
1968	19,770	4,179	99	4,277	216.38	203.94
1969	20,014	4,739	118	4,857	242.68	214.00
1970	20,361	5,125	157	5,281	259.37	215.07
1971	20,742	5,741	150	5,900	284.45	221.53
1972	21,115	6,318	185	6,503	307.98	232.44
1973	23,301	7,057	232	7,289	312.82	227.18
1974	23,978	9,099	272	9,372	390.86	259.71
1975	24,646	11,315	266	11,581	469.89	278.70
1976	25,312	13,340	339	13,679	540.42	292.59
1977	26,094	15,737	283	16,619	636.89	314.67
1978	26,777	17,682	496	18,178	678.87	309.42
1979	27,459	20,623	450	21,073	767.44	319.63
1980	27,500	25,064	512	25,577	930.07	348.08
1981	28,100	30,342	384	30,726	1,093.45	370.54

Source: Board of Trustees, Federal Hospital Insurance Trust Fund, *1982 Annual Report* (Washington, D.C.: Government Printing Office, 1982), table 6, p. 29; *Social Security Bulletin: Annual Statistical Supplement, 1977–79,* pp. 202–3; and our calculations.

[a] As of July 1 of the year. Totals in 1973 and after include pre-65 disability recipients.

[b] Total disbursement divided by number of enrollees.

[c] Nominal insurance deflated by the medical component of the CPI.

actual access to health care. This report is unable to estimate these differential values. Rather, Tables 5.6 and 5.7 report the average nominal and real insurance values of HI and SMI using the methodology described above. Table 5.6 indicates that the nominal insurance value of health insurance rose from $242.68 in 1969 to $1,093.43 in 1981. The increase in insurance rose more rapidly than the rise in the medical component of the CPI, so that real benefits from the hospital insurance program increased by 73 percent over this period. The increase in real benefits for supplementary medical insurance was less uniform, but comparing 1981 to 1969 shows an increase in real benefits of more than 140 percent.

Because the basic coverage of medicare has changed relatively little since 1965, increases in expenditures stem from growth in the elderly population, increased use of services per person, and increases in the costs of services. Although medicare does not have an explicit indexing formula, the promise of a level of services to eligible persons produces an implicit indexing of the value of benefits. The increase in real insurance value per person shown in Tables 5.6 and 5.7 is the result of health costs rising more rapidly than the CPI and the greater use of health services by the elderly population.

TABLE 5.7. Supplementary Medical Insurance: Number of Beneficiaries and Level of Benefits, 1966–81

Year	No. of Enrollees[a] (Thousands)	Total Premiums (Millions)	Per Person Monthly	Disbursements (Millions)			Nominal Insurance Value[b]	Real Insurance Value[c]
				Benefits	Administrative Expenditures	Total Disbursements		
1966	17,736	322	$3.00	$ 128	$ 75	$ 203	$ 37.28	$ 37.28
1967	17,893	640	3.00	1,197	110	1,307	46.26	43.60
1968	18,805	832	4.00	1,518	183	1,702	59.76	52.70
1969	19,195	914	4.00	1,865	196	2,061	56.99	47.26
1970	19,584	1,096	5.30	1,975	238	2,212	53.82	41.92
1971	19,975	1,302	5.30	2,117	260	2,377	50.54	38.14
1972	20,351	1,382	5.60	2,325	290	2,614	57.53	41.78
1973	22,491	1,550	5.80	2,526	318	2,844	89.81	59.67
1974	21,422	1,804	6.30	3,318	410	3,728	117.55	69.72
1975	23,964	1,918	6.70	4,273	462	4,735	144.71	78.35
1976	24,614	2,060	6.70	5,080	542	5,622	167.88	82.94
1977	25,364	2,247	7.20	6,038	467	6,505	202.69	92.38
1978	26,074	2,470	7.70	7,252	503	7,755	244.65	101.90
1979	26,757	2,719	8.20	8,708	557	9,265	303.84	113.71
1980	27,100	3,011	8.70	10,635	610	11,245	373.41	126.54
1981	27,600	3,722	9.60	13,113	915	14,028		

Source: Board of Trustees, Federal Supplementary Medical Insurance Trust Fund, *1982 Annual Report* (Washington, D.C.: Government Printing Office, 1982), table 1, p. 8, and table 6, p. 21; *Social Security Bulletin: Annual Statistical Supplement, 1977–79*; p. 202; and our calculations.
a As of July 1 of the year. Totals include eligible disabled persons in 1973 and thereafter.
b (Total disbursement − total premiums) ÷ number of enrollees.
c Nominal insurance value deflated by the CPI medical component.

Several aspects of the medicare program that determine out-of-pocket costs to older persons are explicitly indexed. These include the deductible amount for inpatient hospital care, which rises as the average amount paid per day for inpatient hospital services increases, the premium payments for SMI which increase by no more than the percent by which monthly social security cash benefits increase, and physician charges, which increase only to the extent justified by certain economic indexes reflecting changes in operating expenses of physicians and general earning levels.

The access to medical service inherent in the medicare program produces an implicit indexing that raises nominal benefit levels when prices rise. The explicit indexing of the cost to individuals results in increases in out-of-pocket costs. When the cost of health care rises more rapidly than the CPI, the real cost (as measured by nominal dollar expenditures deflated by the CPI) will rise. Evidence of this is that the real out-of-pocket cost for health spending by the elderly was 25 percent higher in 1977 than in 1966. However, this individual cost of health care declined as a percentage of the elderly's average income from 15 percent to 12 percent during this period (U.S. Congressional Research Service, 1981, p. 375).

The magnitude of in-kind health transfers is one of the primary reasons Chapter 8 is devoted exclusively to a detailed examination of the consumption of health care services. The provision of subsidized health insurance for the elderly clearly alters the market price for medical services and would be expected to influence consumption of these services.

Food Stamp Program

The food-purchasing power of low-income elderly households is increased by the food stamp program (FSP). Nearly 23 percent of all households participating in the food stamp program in August 1980 contained at least one individual 60 or more years of age (Hiemstra, 1981). This group of households represented around 9 percent of all persons served by the program and received 11 percent of all FSP benefits. Overall, slightly less than 1.9 million of the 10.6 million food stamp participants in August 1980 were 60 or more years of age. The average monthly benefit for participating elderly households was $43. On a per-person basis, benefits for elderly participants were approximately 16 percent below the average for other households in 1980. Slightly over 20 percent of the participating elderly households reported receiving the minimum benefit of $10 per month for one- and two-person households rather than a lesser amount, to which they would have been entitled based solely on their income and household size.

The food stamp program is an outgrowth of pilot programs initiated in the 1960s as alternatives to direct distribution of commodities to low-income households. The food stamp program provides participants additional purchasing power in terms of stamps that are used in place of money to purchase food at retail grocery stores or seeds and plants to grow food for home use. In 1973 all states, as well as Puerto Rico, Guam, and the Virgin Islands, were mandated to implement the program by mid-1974.

A significant program modification introduced by the 1977 Food Stamp Act was the elimination of the purchase requirement. This change resulted in a significant increase in program participation, particularly among the elderly. Prior to this change, participants were required to exchange varying amounts of money for stamps, which could be used to purchase food. The difference between the value of the stamps and the purchase requirement was called the bonus amount, which represented a gross increase in a household's purchasing power for food. The net increase in a household's food purchasing power was somewhat less than the bonus value because of time and out-of-pocket costs incurred in obtaining the stamps. A few states automatically add the value of food stamp benefits directly to SSI payments; in these cases, SSI recipients are ineligible to participate in the food stamp program.

The monthly value of stamps allocated to participating households depends on a number of household characteristics. The value of benefits is determined by reducing the maximum amount of benefits for a given size household by 30 cents for each $1 of net household income derived from earned and unearned sources.

Values of the various components that determine benefits as well as eligibility criteria have been legislatively revised numerous times. The maximum amount of benefits varies with household size and is determined by the U.S. Department of Agriculture's thrifty food plan. The purpose of the thrifty food plan is to estimate sufficient quantities of food to provide nutritionally adequate diets for households of particular sizes and compositions. The plan is repriced monthly, and food stamp benefits have been periodically adjusted to reflect these cost increases. Food stamp benefits levels were increased by 11.5 percent as of January 1, 1981, to reflect the increase in the costs of the thrifty food plan between September 1979 and September 1980, and again in October 1982 to reflect the increase in food prices from September 1980 through June 30, 1982, less 1 percent. Subsequent adjustments scheduled for October 1, 1983, and October 1, 1984, are to reflect price changes in the twelve months ending the preceding June, less 1 percent. Prior to the 1980 amendments to the Food Stamp Act, semiannual adjustments in benefit levels occurred based on the rate of increase in the thrifty food plan.

Eligibility requirements for older persons to participate in the food stamp program involve an income test as well as a limitation on assets. The asset eligibility limitation includes the amount of cash, savings accounts, stocks and bonds, and value of vacation homes. The total value of these items cannot exceed $3,000 if one of the household members is 60 years of age or older. Net income, which is calculated by subtracting some types of household expenditures from gross income, determines the proportion of the maximum benefit participating households are entitled to receive. For each additional dollar of net income, benefits are reduced by 30 cents. Thus, a net income of approximately three times the cost of the thrifty food plan for any given size household is required to reduce benefits to the minimum amount of $10 per month for one- or two-person households.

In order to consider the impact that inflation has on elderly FSP participants, it is necessary to consider two effects: the effect of inflation on eligibility for the program and the effect of inflation on benefit levels of those who do participate. Furthermore, in each instance it is necessary to separate effects into short-run and long-run components. The short-run effects occur during intervals between legislative and automatic adjustments in program rules or benefit levels. Longer-run effects relate to how the legislative and periodic adjustments in program rules or benefits compare to the rate of change in prices.

In general, adjustments in the way the program has operated over the last decade imply an increase in real benefits per person of slightly over 40 percent (see Table 5.8). Although these values represent the benefits to participants of all ages, it seems likely that real benefits for the elderly have changed in a similar fashion.

Inflation would generally be expected to reduce participation levels in the short run as nominal incomes rise, and the eligibility standards and benefit formula remain unchanged. This would mean fewer eligible households for a given set of poverty income guidelines. As poverty guidelines are adjusted periodically to reflect price level changes over time, some or all of the short-run losses in eligibility could be eliminated. Over the last decade, increases in the number of participants indicates that adjustments in program rules have

TABLE 5.8. Average Monthly Food Stamp Benefits per Person, 1970–81

Fiscal Year	Current Value	Real Value[a]
1970	$10.55	$ 9.44
1971	13.55	11.82
1972	13.48	11.35
1973	14.60	11.35
1974	17.61	11.44
1975	21.41	12.68
1976	23.93	13.35
1977	24.73	13.24
1978	26.83	13.14
1979	30.55	13.28
1980	34.34	14.03
1981[b]	37.89	14.34

Source: Personal communication from Dr. Steve Hiemstra, director of Economic Analysis Division, Food and Nutrition Service, U.S. Department of Agriculture.

[a] Column 2 divided by CPI component for food at home (1967 = 100).

[b] First six months.

more than compensated for any effect of higher gross income due to inflation.

Other In-kind Benefit Programs

The low-income aged are eligible for a variety of in-kind benefit programs, along with social and employment services. These programs include public housing, nutritional programs, employment services through the Comprehensive Employment and Training Act, services provided by the Administration on Aging, and a number of other programs that provide a low level of total benefits. Estimated expenditures for these programs in fiscal year 1982 are shown in Table 5.1.

Most of these programs were introduced during President Lyndon Johnson's War on Poverty years of the 1960s and were expanded during the recession years of the early 1970s. Many are aimed at the poor or the unemployed in general and do not contain age-related eligibility conditions. The aged receive benefits because of their low-income status.

GOVERNMENT TRANSFERS AND THE PURCHASING POWER OF OLDER PERSONS

The economic well-being of older persons is determined by their ability to obtain and consume goods and services. The model developed in Chapters 1 and 2 indicates that in-kind benefits and the flow of services from personal wealth should be added to cash income to derive the purchasing power of the elderly. Our discussion above has illustrated the importance of governmental cash and in-kind transfers for older Americans. Marilyn Moon (1977) estimates that in-kind transfers to the aged average more than 10 percent of the mean current income for aged families. Thomas Borzilleri (1980) attributes even greater importance to such benefits by estimating that they increase mean income of families whose head is aged 65 or older by 14.4 percent and the mean income of single older persons by 32.2 percent. The inclusion of in-kind transfers in the determination of total family resources significantly reduces the degree of inequality among the elderly (Moon, 1977). The in-kind transfers are primarily poverty programs and are therefore targeted at the low-income population. Borzilleri estimates that in-kind benefits raise the mean total income of older persons with less than $7,000 of cash income by 68 percent.

In-kind benefits combined with cash transfers are a major source of income of older persons, especially the low-income elderly. Estimates by the Congressional Budget Office of the effect on the income of low-income elderly in relation to the poverty threshold are shown in Table 5.9. Without the public tax/transfer system and no other changes in income, 59.9 percent of persons 65 and over would have had incomes below the poverty rate.

TABLE 5.9. Families Aged 65 and Older Below the Poverty Level under Alternative Definitions, Fiscal Year 1976

Definition of Income	Families Below Poverty Level	
	Number (Thousands)	Percentage
Pretax/pretransfer income	9,647	59.9
Pretax/post–social insurance income	3,459	21.5
Pretax/post–money transfer income	2,686	16.7
Pretax/post–money and in-kind transfer income	977	6.1
Post-tax/post-total transfer income	982	6.1

Source: U.S. Congressional Budget Office, *Poverty Status of Families Under Alternative Definitions,* Background Paper No. 17, revised (Washington, D.C.: Government Printing Office, 1977), p. 12.

Social insurance income lowered this to 21.5 percent, and other money transfers further reduced the percentage of elderly below the poverty rate to 16.7. The inclusion of in-kind transfers results in an incidence of poverty of only 6 percent. In the absence of these programs, people would adjust life-cycle income and work efforts. In addition, older persons would probably receive increased transfers from family and charitable organizations. Thus, it is unlikely that almost 60 percent of the elderly would be below the poverty line without these programs.

Borzilleri (1980) finds a greater effect of in-kind benefit programs on the purchasing power of low income elderly. He adjusts the Bureau of Labor Statistics budgets to include the value of medicare and concludes that "virtually the entire aged family population had sufficient income to purchase the lower living standard" (p. 40). Smeeding (1982) finds a smaller poverty reduction effect when he uses the cash equivalent value in utility terms of in-kind benefits (see also Moon 1979).

The significant improvement in the income of the elderly reported in Chapter 4 underestimates the gain in purchasing power of the elderly because of the simultaneous expansion of in-kind benefit programs over the past two decades. We have shown here how these programs, along with cash transfers, respond to price increases. The increased importance of federal transfers in the income of the elderly has done much to insulate older persons from declines in real income due to inflation.

6 Fluctuations in the Real Value of Earnings, Social Security, and Employer Pensions

The primary sources of cash income for older persons are earnings, social security benefits, and employer pension benefits. In Chapter 4 we saw that earnings decline in importance with age as the average time spent working is reduced, while social security and pension benefits become increasingly important with retirement. In examining the income patterns of the past several decades, we must give careful consideration to changes in behavior from one cohort of older persons to the next and also to the development of the benefit programs during this time. A second set of issues relates to how inflation can be expected to influence the real income of older persons within the legal and economic framework prevailing during the early 1980s. In this chapter we seek to identify these effects by focusing on the changes in the real value of earnings, social security benefits, and employer pension benefits and by examining each of these sources for trends in real value and the manner in which income responds to increases in consumer prices. This helps explain the findings on the change in real income during the 1970s reported in Chapter 4.

EARNINGS, AGING, AND INFLATION

Life-cycle Patterns of Work

Individuals develop life-cycle plans for time and resource allocation that generate anticipated age-earnings patterns. As persons age, they tend to reduce their labor supply either by entirely leaving the labor force or by working fewer hours. Table 6.1 uses male age-specific labor force participation rates to illustrate this point. For example, the 1982 rates decline continuously with increasing age as a larger proportion of men are out of the labor force with each additional year of age. Average hours per week of those working also tend to decline with increasing age.

Reductions in the amount or length of work typically will result in decreased earnings. Thus, the declines in mean cohort earnings reported in Chapter 4 are not unexpected and should not be considered purely a response to inflation. Instead they represent, to a large degree, anticipated declines in earnings in response to reduced labor supply with age. This reduction in

TABLE 6.1. Labor Force Participation Rates: Males by Age, 1968–82

Age	1968	1970	1975	1979	1980	1981	1982
55	91.9%	91.7%	87.5%	85.9%	84.9%	84.8%	86.4%
56	91.2	90.7	85.7	84.2	83.0	82.6	84.0
57	90.6	89.1	84.4	81.8	81.5	80.9	80.8
58	88.8	87.7	83.6	80.3	80.9	80.0	79.9
59	86.6	87.5	80.3	78.8	78.6	77.4	77.9
60	84.8	84.0	76.9	73.5	73.9	73.2	72.1
61	82.8	81.2	73.5	70.3	69.6	68.1	67.1
62	76.4	73.9	64.4	60.1	56.8	54.4	54.3
63	71.9	69.4	58.2	53.7	52.3	48.2	45.2
64	69.0	64.4	53.0	49.4	48.8	45.0	44.2
65	53.4	50.0	38.7	36.9	35.0	33.3	30.6
66	46.6	44.7	33.6	31.6	30.4	29.0	28.9
67	40.8	39.4	30.4	26.2	27.9	28.0	27.1
68	37.5	37.7	28.5	26.3	24.1	25.0	24.8
69	33.9	34.0	25.8	24.8	22.8	22.1	22.6
70	30.2	30.2	23.7	23.8	21.3	18.9	21.3
71	25.5	27.9	22.4	20.2	19.0	18.0	16.2
72	24.5	24.8	22.6	17.8	16.0	16.5	15.4
73	21.6	22.6	19.8	19.1	14.9	15.5	16.0
74	20.0	19.1	15.9	15.8	16.5	14.0	13.6
75+	12.6	12.0	10.2	8.7	8.8	9.0	8.5

Source: Unpublished data from U.S. Bureau of Labor Statistics.
Note: The labor force participation rate is the percentage of the population group that is employed or looking for work.

market work also explains the increasing importance of social security and pension benefits to older persons.

Table 6.1 also shows a substantial decline in the age-specific participation rates of men from 1968 to 1982. These declines are the result of a greater proportion of older males choosing to be out of the labor force at each age. This observation is very significant when examining the trend in the income of older persons during the 1970s. For example, the average earnings of all men aged 65 and over would be expected to fall during this period as a smaller proportion of older men are working. The finding that the real cash income of this group does not fall is significant and implies a growing importance of transfer income during this period. The growth in cash income will also understate the improvement in well-being because of the simultaneous increase in time away from work implied by the data in Table 6.1.

Inflation and Labor Force Participation

Within the framework of planned reductions in labor supply, unanticipated events such as unexpectedly high rates of inflation may cause persons to change their lifetime plans for work and retirement. These changes would occur in response to changes in the real wage rate and to shifts in the real value of a person's wealth portfolio.

As long as real wages and real wealth are unchanged in response to inflation, older persons would not modify their work and retirement plans during periods of rising prices. The important concept is how inflation alters the real wage and wealth that a person expected. Clearly, the hourly wage may change in late life even without price changes. Wage rates change in response to economy-wide productivity gains, other macroeconomic conditions, individuals augmenting their skills, or persons suffering declines in their talents, perhaps for health reasons. Life-cycle models usually predict declining real wages during the final work years.

In general, economists would argue that the real wage would be unaffected by inflation, that is, that the nominal wage rises at the same rate as prices. However, various institutional arrangements such as labor contracts and equal opportunity laws may limit wage adjustments. These same institutions may preclude reductions in nominal wage rates but allow real wage reductions. Thus some employers may wish to lower the wage of their older employees but are unable to do so in nominal terms. Inflation permits firms to lower real wages and encourage earlier retirement.

Other potential labor supply responses to inflation could be caused by changes in real wealth. Greater wealth increases the tendency of older workers to withdraw from the labor force. Thus, if inflation lowers the real value of wealth, older persons will be more inclined to remain in the labor force and less likely to retire. The evidence in Chapter 4 did not indicate that the assets of the elderly were particularly vulnerable to declines in real value in response to inflation.

Work and Earnings for the RHS Couples

To examine changes in earnings, a sample of all husbands and wives who remained together from 1969 to 1975 is selected from the Retirement History Survey. All persons with reported hourly wage rates of below $1 or in excess of $50 are deleted from the sample to prevent those extreme values from affecting the analysis. During this period, these couples age and economic conditions change. Table 6.2 shows that the labor force participation rate for husbands falls from 79.4 to 25.2 percent. For men in the labor force, average hours of work decline from 42.6 to 34.4 hours per week. Less significant declines for wives in both these measures of labor supply are reported. These reductions in labor supply reflect expected declines in work with age and any response to inflation and other economic events.

During this period, average earnings for all men in the sample decline by more than 57 percent, reflecting reduced market work. The earnings of the wives fall by 23 percent. These declines in nominal earnings occur despite rising nominal wages. The average wage of working men rose by one-third, from $3.71 in 1969 to $4.93 in 1975. The mean wage of working wives rose by

TABLE 6.2. Labor Supply of Couples in Retirement History Study, 1969–75

	Husbands		Wives	
Year	Labor Force Participation	Hours per Week[a]	Labor Force Participation	Hours per Week[a]
1969	79.4%	42.6	33.1%	35.9
1971	65.1	41.3	31.7	35.8
1973	40.5	39.4	25.5	34.9
1975	25.2	34.4	20.1	32.9

Source: Retirement History Study, 1969–75 interviews.
Note: The labor force participation rate is the percentage of the population group that is employed or looking for work.
[a] Average hours per week of those working in each year.

TABLE 6.3. Real Wage and Earnings of Couples in RHS, 1969–75

	Husbands		Wives	
Year	Average Wage	Mean Earnings	Average Wage	Mean Earnings
1969	$3.38	$6,181	$2.00	$1,383
1971	3.33	5,240	2.14	1,260
1973	3.35	3,546	2.18	1,010
1975	3.06	1,808	2.19	725

Source: Retirement History Study, 1969–75 interviews.
Note: Values in 1967 dollars.

60 percent. The nominal wage for these older men rose at a slower rate than the CPI. Thus, their real wage fell by almost 10 percent and average real earnings dropped by 70 percent. By contrast, the real wage of the wives rose by 10 percent (see Table 6.3), but real earnings fell because of reductions in labor supply.

If this decline in real wages were entirely attributable to inflation, the participation rate of these older men will have fallen because of the inflation-reduced real wage. The magnitude of reduced work effort depends on the responsiveness of labor supply to changes in the real wage. Most studies find that older men and women increase their labor supply in response to higher wage rates (Clark and Barker, 1981). Thus, declines in real wage rates attributable to inflation would tend to reduce market work of older persons. For a detailed discussion of the retirement decision of the RHS couples, see Clark and Johnson (1980); the hours-of-work decision is studied in Clark, Gohmann, and Sumner (1981).

All the decline in the real wage should not be attributed to inflation. As noted above, wage rates may decline as older persons attempt to reduce their weekly hours. Clark, Gohmann, and Sumner (1981) find that the hourly wage rate falls significantly as hours per week of work are reduced. Gustman and Steinmeier (1981) show that real wages for older workers do not fall as long as workers remain on their career jobs, but that real wages do drop if the person attempts to shift to part-time employment. Thus, the decline in real wage rates is in part a response to the decision of older persons to reduce their work efforts.

REAL VALUE OF SOCIAL SECURITY BENEFITS

The real value of social security benefits over time is determined by the rate of inflation and the rate of increase in these benefits. Throughout the first three decades of the system, benefits were increased periodically by specific congressional action. The 1972 amendments provided for full automatic indexing of benefits after retirement starting in 1975. Past earnings records were indexed to provide for rising real initial benefits. These changes were described in detail in Chapter 5.

Table 6.4 shows the percentage increase in the primary insurance amount (PIA) and the consumer price index for the decade of the RHS cohort. Persons receive 100 percent of their PIA if they retire at age 65. Early retirement reduces initial benefits, and delayed retirement increases them. In most cases, increases in the PIA after retirement can be translated into similar increases in actual benefits. Table 6.4 indicates that for a person retired in 1967, benefits would have risen by 245 percent between 1968 and 1982. Since the CPI rose by only 179 percent, real social security benefits have increased by approx-

TABLE 6.4. Percentage Increases in Primary Insurance Amount and CPI, 1968–82

Year	Annual		Cumulative[a]	
	PIA[b]	CPI[c]	PIA	CPI
1968	13.0	4.2	13	4.2
1969	0.0	5.4	13	9.8
1970	15.0	5.9	30	16.3
1971	10.0	4.3	43	21.3
1972	20.0	3.3	43	25.3
1973	0.0	6.2	72	33.1
1974	11.0	11.0	72	47.7
1975	8.0	9.1	90	61.2
1976	6.4	5.8	106	70.5
1977	5.9	6.4	119	81.5
1978	6.5	7.6	132	95.3
1979	9.9	11.5	147	117.7
1980	14.2	13.5	171	147.0
1981	11.2	10.2	210	172.3
1982	7.4	3.9	245	179.0

Source: *Social Security Bulletin: Annual Statistical Supplement, 1977–1979,* p. 26; recent issues of the *Social Security Bulletin,* and Chapter 3.

[a] Measured from 1968 to year.

[b] Increases awarded at various times throughout the year.

[c] Annual increase, measured from January to December.

TABLE 6.5. Social Security Benefits in January of Each Year, as a Percentage of Initial Benefits, 1968–82

Year	1968	1969	1970	1971	1972	1973	1974	1975	1976	1977	1978	1979	1980	1981	1982
1968	100.0	113.0	130.0	143.0	143.0	172.0	172.0	190.0	206.0	219.0	232.0	247.0	271.0	310.0	345.0
1969		100.0	115.0	127.0	127.0	152.0	152.0	168.0	182.0	194.0	205.0	218.0	240.0	274.0	305.0
1970			100.0	110.0	110.0	132.0	132.0	147.0	158.0	168.0	178.0	190.0	209.0	239.0	266.0
1971				100.0	100.0	120.0	120.0	133.0	144.0	153.0	162.0	173.0	190.0	217.0	241.0
1972					100.0	120.0	120.0	133.0	144.0	153.0	162.0	173.0	190.0	217.0	241.0
1973						100.0	100.0	111.0	120.0	128.0	135.0	144.0	158.0	181.0	201.0
1974							100.0	111.0	120.0	128.0	135.0	144.0	158.0	181.0	201.0
1975								100.0	108.0	115.0	122.0	130.0	142.0	162.0	180.0
1976									100.0	106.4	113.0	120.0	132.0	151.0	168.0
1977										100.0	105.9	113.0	124.0	142.0	158.0
1978											100.0	106.5	117.0	134.0	149.0
1979												100.0	109.9	126.0	140.0
1980													100.0	114.3	127.0
1981														100.0	111.2
1982															100.0

Source: Social Security Bulletin: Annual Statistical Supplement, 1977–1979, p. 26; recent issues of Social Security Bulletin.
Note: The values along a row indicate the social security benefit in each year as a percentage of benefits in the year a person retired. For example, find the year of retirement on the left-hand column, say 1971. In 1974, the benefit for a person who retired in 1971 is 120 percent of the initial benefit received in 1971. These percentages represent the minimum percentage increase in primary insurance amounts.

72

imately 25 percent. Table 6.5 shows the cumulative increase between the year of retirement and 1982 for subsequent retirees. The trend in the real value of benefits beginning in any year can be determined by dividing the information in Table 6.5 by the corresponding CPI data shown in Chapter 3.

Retirees have not suffered any loss in the real value of their incomes through changes in social security benefits. In fact, persons already receiving benefits in the late 1960s have had the real value of their benefits increase over the last decade. Most of the real increase occurred between 1968 and 1972, prior to the automatic adjustment of benefits. Since that time, benefits have risen in step with increases in the CPI, and the real value of benefits should by and large have remained constant.

The social security benefits for new retirees were also rising during the 1970s. Table 6.6 shows the increase in initial benefits for 65-year-olds with average monthly earnings (AME) of $250 to $1,000. The benefit for each AME increased by more than the increase in the CPI rise. Thus the real initial social security benefits for persons with average monthly earnings of between $250 and $1,000 rose by 10 to 35 percent during this decade. The AME is usually rising for successive cohorts of retirees, and as a result average initial benefits rose by more than the increase indicated in Table 6.6.

This examination of increases in social security benefits after retirement indicates that real social security income was largely insulated from erosion by price increases. The ad hoc and subsequent automatic increases in postretirement benefits were sufficient to stabilize or increase real benefits during this decade. Initial benefits were also rising more rapidly than the rate of inflation. These findings have important implications for the impact of infla-

TABLE 6.6. Benefits for Persons Starting Payments at Age 65 in Various Years When Average Monthly Earnings Are $250, $500, $750, and $1,000, 1969–79

Year	Average Monthly Earnings			
	$250	$500	$750	$1,000
1969	$114.51	$177.51	$218.00[a]	$218.00[a]
1970	131.68	209.13	250.70[a]	250.70[a]
1971	144.85	224.56	295.40[a]	295.40[a]
1972	144.85	224.56	295.40[a]	295.40[a]
1973	173.82	269.46	354.97	404.50[a]
1974	192.93	299.10	394.01	449.54
1975[b]	208.37	323.03	425.53	485.48
1976[b]	221.69	343.66	452.73	516.50
1977[b]	234.77	363.94	479.454	547.00
1978[b]	250.03	387.60	510.62	582.57
1979[b]	274.78	425.60	561.18	640.25

Source: Derived from information in *Social Security Bulletin: Annual Statistical Supplement, 1977–1979*, pp. 15–19.

[a] Reached or exceeded the maximum level of PIA.

[b] Law was effective in June of the given year.

tion on the well-being of the elderly. First, this important component of income of older persons does not decline with price increases. Since over 90 percent of persons aged 65 and over receive social security benefits, this is a significant observation. Second, low-income persons rely more heavily on social security benefits since they do not tend to have other forms of cash income. For example, the 1970 Survey of Newly Entitled Beneficiaries indicated that for the lowest-income groups (those with approximately $1,000 in annual income) social security benefits accounted for over 80 percent of total cash income; however, this proportion drops to less than 20 percent for high-income groups. Also, Upp (1983) reported that 59 percent of all elderly households received at least half their total income from social security benefits; of households actually receiving benefits, 26 percent received 90 percent or more of their total income from social security. This suggests that the real value of incomes of the low-income elderly is more protected against inflation than the income of high-income older persons.

Social security benefits are guaranteed to an eligible person for the remainder of his or her life, and survivor benefits are available for surviving spouses. This lifetime flow of benefits can be viewed as a form of wealth, and its value will depend on the individual's life expectancy. For many people, social security wealth is their largest asset at retirement. Current legislation provides for automatic cost-of-living increases so that the real value of this asset is unaffected by inflation. Whether one views social security as a flow of income or as an asset, it plays a major role in the determination of the well-being of most older persons, and these benefits have not been adversely affected by inflation.

REAL VALUE OF PENSION BENEFITS

The real value of pension benefits during retirement is determined by the rate of inflation and the extent of any postretirement benefit increases. The effect of inflation for a person who initially retires with a 100 percent replacement ratio and receives no increase in benefits can be shown by deflating the nominal benefit. A relatively mild 3 percent inflation rate lowers the real replacement ratio to 86 percent after five years and 75 percent after ten years. By contrast, a 10 percent inflation rate reduces the real replacement rate to 62 percent in only five years.

Another method of illustrating the effect of inflation on the real value of pension benefits is to calculate the expected wealth value of a constant benefit over the person's life. In this formulation, the value of the pension annuity is discounted by an interest rate and the probability of remaining alive to receive the benefit (see Clark and McDermed, 1982). For a 60-year-old male retiree, a 7 percent annual rate of inflation lowers the discounted value of his pension benefit by 43 percent, and a 12 percent inflation rate reduces pension wealth by 58 percent.

These illustrations are made assuming that pension benefits are not increased after a person retires and begins receiving benefits. Many public pension plans are automatically indexed to the rate of inflation, so that benefits rise when the consumer price index increases. The federal civil service retirement system has been fully indexed since 1962. Thus a 10 percent increase in prices over the year leads to a 10 percent increase in retirement benefits. Several other federal retirement programs are similarly indexed (U.S. Congressional Research Service, 1981).

State and local pension plans generally provide for automatic increases but are typically less generous, with many plans limiting increases in any one year to 3 percent or less (Munnell, 1979; Tilove, 1976). Results of a survey of almost 12,000 state and local plans indicate that automatic increases were provided in 23 percent of the plans covering 50 percent of the participants. Most of these increases were subject to some limitation or "cap." Many large plans also provided ad hoc increases. Cook (1981) finds that thirty-four out of sixty-five large public retirement systems covering institutions of higher education provided for automatic CPI-related benefit increases and that all these plans placed limits on the increase. The smaller public plans are less likely to incorporate postretirement benefit increases into their pension plans. Strate (1982) estimates that state pension plans raised benefits of their retirees by 19 to 25 percent between 1974 and 1980. During this period, the CPI rose by 68 percent.

Private pension plans are much less likely to have automatic indexation of pension benefits. Three surveys of large firms indicate that less than 5 percent of private plans provide automatic increases in benefits (Bankers Trust [1980]; Hay Associates [1981]; Hewitt Associates [1981]). The lack of automatic indexation does not mean that benefits are not increased in the private sector. A summary of the three surveys suggests that approximately two-thirds of these large pension plans provided one or more ad hoc increases during the last half of the 1970s (see King, 1982). Table 6.7 describes the type of increases in each of the three surveys. The Bankers Trust and Hewitt Associates surveys find that only 13 percent of all the firms in the two surveys granted more than two increases during the sample periods.

Using data collected by the U.S. Department of Labor, Clark, Allen, and Sumner (1983) find that between 1973 and 1979 average pension benefits for persons already receiving benefits in 1973 increased by 24 percent during a period when the CPI rose by 63 percent. Benefit increases were far more prevalent in large plans than in smaller plans. All plans with more than 10,000 recipients awarded at least one increase, and almost one-quarter of these plans granted benefit increases each year. In contrast, only 16 percent of plans with less than 100 recipients awarded any increases.

TABLE 6.7. Types of Postretirement Pension Adjustments — Private Pension Plans (Percentage of Plans Surveyed, Number of Plans in Parentheses)

Type of Adjustment	Hay Associates, 1981[a]		Bankers Trust, 1975–79		Hewitt Associates, 1975–81	
Total	100.0%	(417)	100.0%	(216)	100.0%	(117)
No adjustments during period surveyed	44.0%	(183)	25.0%	(54)	15.0%	(17)
Ad hoc adjustments during period surveyed	52.0%	(216)	71.0%	(153)	85.0%	(100)
Automatic annual adjustments during period surveyed	4.0%	(18)	4.0%	(9)	—	
Triggered by and related to CPI increases (with a "cap")	3.0%	(12)	4.0%	(9)	—	
Fixed percentage annual increase	1.0%	(5)	—		—	

Sources: Reprinted by permission of *The Gerontologist*/the *Journal of Gerontology* from Francis King, "Indexing Retirement Benefits," *The Gerontologist* 22 (December 1982), p. 492. Data from Hay Associates, "Hay-Huggins Noncash Compensation Comparison" (1981), adjustments during 1981; Bankers Trust, *Corporate Pension Plan Study: A Guide for the 1980s* (1980), adjustments after 1974 to end of 1979; Hewitt Associates, "Post-retirement Pension Increases Among Major U.S. Employers" (1981), adjustments from January 1975 through early 1981.

[a] The above data cover 351 industrial firms and utilities. The study analyzed responses from 198 additional plans, which were classified as financial and service sector plans. Since this "finance/service" category includes some public employee plans, these 198 plans are left out of this table.

These surveys show that the popular notion that employer pension benefits are fixed at retirement is incorrect. Instead, there is a definite pattern of ad hoc and automatic increases. However, these increases generally have been less than increases in consumer prices, and as a result the real value of benefits has fallen after retirement. The following section examines further the change in employer pension benefits after retirement.

Change in Postretirement Pension Benefits, 1968–74

We examined respondents in the Retirement History Study for changes in their pension benefits between 1968 and 1974. Table 6.8 shows the mean real benefit of married men during this period divided by the survey year in which these men first are shown to be receiving benefits. For persons receiving benefits in 1968, the mean real 1974 benefit was 3 percent lower. Somewhat larger declines are observed for the groups that began to receive benefits in 1970 and 1972.

These declines seem small, especially for those who have been retired the longest. This is the result of using the mean as a summary statistic and the fact that some people report large increases in pension benefits from one survey to the next. The pension income of these men may rise because firms

TABLE 6.8. Real Pension Benefits of Married Men in RHS, 1968–74

Year of First Benefit	Real Pension Benefit[a]			
	1968	1970	1972	1974
1968	$2,619[b]	$2,325	$2,341	$2,547
1970		2,159	2,107	2,071
1972			2,220	1,956
1974				1,942

Source: Retirement History Study, 1969–75 interviews.

[a] Benefits are in 1967 dollars and are means.

[b] The 1969 survey did not identify the proportion of family pension income in 1968 attributable to the husband and wife. The 1968 figure represents our estimate based on examination of information in subsequent surveys and on 1969 data on family members receiving pension benefits.

TABLE 6.9. Percentage of Married Men in RHS with Change in Pension Income between Initial Year of Benefits and 1974

Change in Benefit	1968 Retirees	1970 Retirees	1972 Retirees
Any increase in nominal benefits	49.1	52.9	53.2
Loss in real benefits	70.0	64.7	69.0
Gain in real benefits	30.0	35.3	31.0
Above mean benefit			
Loss in real benefits	79.3	78.3	81.4
Gain in real benefits	20.7	21.7	18.6
Below mean benefit			
Loss in real benefit	64.9	57.7	62.1
Gain in real benefits	35.1	42.3	37.9

Source: Retirement History Study, 1969–75 interviews.

have raised their benefits or because they begin to receive a second pension. The addition of a second benefit may substantially raise pension income and have a significant effect on the sample mean.

A more detailed picture of benefit changes is shown in Table 6.9. Only about half the retirees received any nominal increase in their pensions between initial receipt and 1974. Over two-thirds of the sample suffer a loss in their real benefits over the periods. Some 53 percent of 1968 retirees had a decline in real benefits of more than 25 percent by 1974. Of the more recent retirees, 40 percent of those starting benefits in 1970 and 26 percent of those starting benefits in 1972 had a 25 percent or more drop in the real value of their benefits. These declines may not be due solely to inflation. Nominal benefits may be reduced if a person returns to work. Also, some pensions provide supplements for early retirees, which are reduced when the person reaches age 62 or 65 and becomes eligible for social security benefits. The finding that over 20 percent of the men have a 25 percent or larger gain in real benefits between the year of initial benefits and 1974 suggests that some men are adding new pensions.

Fewer wives in the RHS couples have pension benefits, because they are younger than their husbands and have had fewer years of market work. The real value of the wife's benefit declines more during the survey period, probably because the wives worked for firms that were less likely to provide benefit increases and because wives are less likely to have a second pension.

A final observation concerns the change in real value by the level of initial benefits. Table 6.9 shows that when the sample is divided at the mean of initial benefits, a smaller proportion of persons with initial benefits below the mean had the real value of their benefits decline. Further evidence that much of the gain in real pension income can be attributed to starting a second pension is the finding that almost 90 percent of persons with gains of 25 percent or more are persons that had pension income below the mean when they first started receiving benefits. These relatively low benefits were eventually supplemented by retirement income from more recent employment.

These results are generally consistent with the findings of Thompson (1978), who found that the median pension benefit for completely retired pensioners in the RHS aged 63 to 64 rose from $1,980 in 1970 to $2,160 in 1974. This represents a fall in the real value of the benefits, since the CPI increased by 14 percent and the nominal benefits rose by only 9 percent. The use of completely retired persons probably eliminates many who acquired a second pension by continued employment. This restricting of the sample population reduces the variability of pension income over the period and reduces much of the gains in pension income reported above.

Change in Initial Pension Benefits

Benefit formulas for employer pensions vary considerably across the economy. In the private sector, most plans are noncontributory defined benefit plans. In a defined benefit plan, the employer promises to pay a specified benefit to each worker who achieves sufficient job tenure and reaches the age of eligibility for benefits. Typically the employee has some choice concerning retirement, and the annual pension benefit will depend on his or her decision.

The benefit is often determined by multiplying an average salary during final working years by the benefit formula and the number of years of service. In most instances an additional year of work will increase the benefit because of rising wages and increased job tenure. Despite this gain in annual benefits, the discounted expected value of the flow of pension benefits may have fallen. The discounted value of pension benefits may decline because workers give up a year of benefits when they defer retirement after they are eligible for retirement benefits. Thus, net pension compensation for the year of work is equal to present value of the higher benefit minus the year of benefits foregone.

To examine the relationship between continued work and the value of benefits, Clark and McDermed (1982) construct a hypothetical pension benefit formula that approximates many industrial plans. They assume that the salary history is determined over a five-year period and that 1 percent of this average is paid for each year of service. In the absence of price increases, wages rise by 3 percent per year; however, once an individual retires, benefits remain constant. To calculate the expected present value of the flow of earnings and benefits, future income is discounted at a rate of 3 percent. The wealth variables are derived by using mortality rates from the 1971 Group Annuity Mortality Tables for a white male. In this initial comparison, the employee is assumed to have joined the firm at age 45 and is eligible for full pension benefits at age 60. The individual had a beginning annual earnings of $6,000, so that, in the absence of inflation, at the end of his fifteen years of service his salary is $9,076.

On the basis of these assumptions, the individual could retire on an annual pension benefit of $1,284, or 14.7 percent of the previous year's earnings. If prices remained stable throughout the lifetime of the retiree, the expected discounted wealth from the pension benefits would be $16,924. The 60-year-old employee must decide whether to accept this benefit or to work an additional year. Annual earnings from another year of work would be $9,349, which would increase pension benefits beginning in the following year to $1,411. Discounting this flow of benefits to age 60 yields a present value of pension income equal to $17,242. Thus there is a pension wealth gain from continued employment of $318.

As the worker ages, this pension compensation incentive for retirement is altered. Under the assumptions of the model, wages continue to rise at an annual rate of 3 percent, and this increasing wage base generates higher annual pension benefits with continued employment. In this example, this value is shown to change sign at age 63. Thus, prior to age 63 the wage is an underestimate of total compensation; however, continued employment in late life implies that the wage eventually becomes an overestimate of the gain from continued work as the net change in pension wealth becomes negative. The age of this reversal is a function of inflation, tenure, life expectancy, and other employment characteristics.

Inflation will alter the real values of wages and pension benefits only to the extent that the nominal values do not rise to reflect fully the increase in prices. This lack of adjustment may stem from institutional constraints or labor market imperfections. Once a general model of inflationary effects is constructed, specific assumptions concerning the adjustment process can be made. Inflation has the potential for altering nominal and real wages and pension benefits in each period. Price increases also raise the rate by which future nominal income is discounted.

The influence of inflation on the accumulation of pension wealth can be introduced into the analysis by a variety of methods. In the following, prices are assumed to have remained constant throughout a person's work life until the worker considers retiring. At this point, inflation is assumed to rise to a specified level of between 4 and 14 percent and then remain at this new rate. Wages are assumed to rise to reflect inflation fully, while pension benefits are held constant after retirement. As a result, higher rates of inflation have a considerable effect on the value of the benefit stream. The discounted value of pension wealth for the 60-year-old retiree declines from $16,924 with no inflation to $9,470 with inflation at a 7 percent annual rate, whereas if prices continued to rise at a 14 percent rate, the wealth value declines to $6,350. Comparable declines are registered in pension wealth regardless of age of retirement. This reduction in pension wealth as a result of inflation will tend to delay retirement by workers eligible for pension benefits.

If the individual continues to be employed, his nominal wage by assumption rises by the rate of inflation. Thus the real wage is invariate with respect to price changes. The nominal pension benefit rises after the additional year of work because of the higher nominal wage in the last period. The mechanism of the inflation effect on initial nominal benefits is as follows: Inflation raises last period wages, higher wages increase the average salary, thus raising the benefits over what they would have been without inflation. In the present example, we have assumed that the inflation began in the last year of work. Therefore, a comparison between rates of inflation alters the wage only in this last period. Because of the length of the salary-averaging period (five years), annual benefits at age 61 do not rise sufficiently to offset fully the increase in prices during the previous year. Therefore, the annual accumulation of real pension benefits is reduced with a change in the rate of inflation.

The change in pension wealth from an additional year of work in the absence of inflation was illustrated earlier. In the model, this compensation effect of pension coverage was found to be positive between the ages of 60 and 62 and negative thereafter. The introduction of inflation significantly alters the net accumulation of pension wealth from continued employment. An inflation rate of 4 percent is sufficient to make the pension compensation effect negative as soon as the individual becomes eligible to receive benefits at age 60. Thus the existence of inflation lowers total annual compensation. The combination of inflation and aging effects produces a loss in pension wealth from continued employment by 10 percent or more by the late sixties. A worker's total compensation falls as the rate of inflation increases because of the pension wealth effect described above.

This decline in real compensation in response to inflation may influence the retirement decision. By examining a model of pension benefits and earnings, two distinct effects of inflation on workers who are covered by an employer pension can be identified. First, there is a large wealth effect if benefits are not adjusted with inflation. At age 60, a 7 percent rate of inflation for the rest of one's life reduces the value of pension wealth by 44 percent, while a 14 percent inflation results in a decline of 62 percent. This wealth effect would increase the likelihood that people will remain in the labor force and delay retirement.

The compensation effect is more complex and is a function of a number of pension characteristics, so one should be more cautious in generalizing the results. In the example derived in this section, however, an inflation rate of 7 percent reduces total compensation by 5 percent for those in their early sixties and by 2 percent for those in their late sixties. Economic theory states that compensation changes have both income and substitution effects, and as a result the qualitative influence is ambiguous and a subject for empirical research. Although empirical studies differ in their findings, our own research using older workers from the Retirement History Study indicates that people increase their work time in response to wage increases. Thus, a reduction in the annual compensation because of inflation would tend to reduce hours of work and encourage earlier retirement.

This example illustrates the effect of inflation on pension compensation and wealth when benefits are not increased after retirement. It is important to recall the evidence reported earlier. In contrast to the assumptions of the example in this section, wages rose by less than prices during the 1970s, while nominal pension benefits were raised by employers. In addition, social security benefits were rising by a rate equal to CPI increases. Thus, in some cases older workers were faced with declining real wages if they remained employed, but would have had benefits rising with prices if they retired. Persons in this situation become increasingly likely to retire.

The three primary sources of income for older persons are examined in this chapter for their responsiveness to price changes. In Chapter 4, earnings, social security, and pension benefits are shown to account for 94 percent of average family cash income in 1968 for couples in the Retirement History Study, and 87 percent in 1974. During this period earnings decline in importance while social security and pension income increase. An understanding of these income sources will to a large measure explain the income-inflation relationship for the elderly. Our review indicates that the primary income sources of the elderly are not fixed in nominal terms but instead respond to price fluctuations. This helps explain the improvement in the real income of the elderly during the inflationary past decade as noted in Chapter 4. The general economic relationships and institutional responses outlined above will also be useful in Chapter 9 in investigating the effects of inflation in the coming years.

7 Expenditure Patterns of the Elderly

Individuals devote different amounts of their resources to the purchase of specific commodities. The model described in Chapters 1 and 2 indicates that expenditures are a function of income, prices, and individual preferences. In this chapter, we explore the variation in expenditure patterns of elderly households, along with changes in purchases during selected time periods, and examine the limited time series evidence to determine the effect of inflation on the changing expenditures of the elderly. We begin with an evaluation of the alternative sources of data in this analysis.

ALTERNATIVE DATA SOURCES FOR EXPENDITURE ANALYSIS

The most recent available Consumer Expenditure Survey (CES) was conducted by the Bureau of Labor Statistics in 1972–73. Its objective was to collect information to update the consumer price index. The survey consisted of two parts: (1) a diary portion in which respondents kept a record of selected expenditures for two-week periods, and (2) an interview panel in which households reported information every three months. The interview component covered the 1972 and 1973 years, with each year including approximately 10,000 different households. In this survey both unrelated individuals and families were considered households.

Approximately 3,600 families in the sample each year had a head of household 55 years of age and older, the age group of special interest to our study. Since both years were parts of the same survey, most tabulations of these data combine data from the two years. For example, budget shares for various subgroups of the elderly reported by Barnes and Zedlewski (1981) are based on the combined data set. For our purposes, we had a special interest in how expenditure differences between the two years may have been influenced by price increases. Even though the data for the two years involve households with similar characteristics, contrasts must be interpreted cautiously since the same households are not observed in each year. Because the data set is very comprehensive with respect to detailed expenditure information, it provides a valuable benchmark for determining which subgroups of households would be most affected by differential changes in relative prices accompanying inflation. Also, it makes it possible to compare expenditures in order to identify potential price changes that may be especially important to the elderly.

TABLE 7.1. Average Expenditures and Budget Shares by Age of Household Head, 1972–73 CES

Expenditure Category	Age of Household Head					
	Under 55 Years			55 and Older		
Food, alcohol, tobacco		$2,093.82	17.1%		$1,554.19	18.9%
a. Food	$1,854.60			$1,414.39		
b. Alcohol	90.72			46.67		
c. Tobacco	148.51			93.13		
Housing		2,749.22	22.4		1,801.87	21.9
a. Shelter	$1,538.42			909.62		
b. Fuel and utilities	423.81			382.87		
c. Other	786.99			509.38		
Apparel		775.93	6.3		420.09	5.1
Transportation		1,855.00	15.1		1,089.72	13.2
Health and personal care		560.78	4.6		596.01	7.2
Recreation		1,001.88	8.2		613.79	7.5
Insurance and pensions		895.73	7.3		448.58	5.4
Gifts and contributions		369.96	3.0		524.26	6.4
Taxes		1,970.38	16.0		1,188.64	14.4
Totals		$12,272.71	100.0%		$8,237.15	100.0%

Source: Calculated from data in *Consumer Expenditure Survey Series: Interview Survey, 1972–73,* U.S. Department of Labor, Report No. 455–4, 1977, table 5.

The Retirement History Study is the other large data set used in this study. As noted in Chapter 4, this information was collected by the Social Security Administration and initially included slightly over 11,000 respondents between 58 and 63 years of age in 1969. By surveying this sample every two years, a longitudinal data set of information was compiled for a sample of elderly households. We used the information collected in 1969, 1971, 1973, and 1975. By observing the same set of households over time, one can notice changes in expenditure patterns in response to inflation and other factors. Unfortunately, the expenditure information is not as comprehensive as that made available by the CES, and there are some differences in the types of information collected in various years.

CES EXPENDITURE DIFFERENCES BETWEEN THE ELDERLY AND NONELDERLY

Total expenditures for the group of households with heads 55 years of age and older included in the Consumer Expenditure Survey were approximately one-third smaller than those of younger households (see Table 7.1). This was about the same as the relative difference in total income for the two groups of households reported in Chapter 4. The younger group's total expenditures were approximately 96 percent of the total income. The proportion for the 55 and over group was 92 percent. Thus, households of the elderly apparently were saving a little larger share of their incomes than younger households. The corresponding proportion for the 65 and older group was 94 percent, implying a decrease in savings rate as more of the elderly leave the labor force.

There was more similarity between the two age groups in the way expenditures were allocated among categories than was the case for various sources of income discussed in Chapter 4. The elderly allocated a slightly larger share of total expenditures to food, health and personal care, and gifts and contributions relative to the younger group. The elderly had a slightly higher proportion of total expenditures allocated to the food category, even though they spent nearly $540 less than younger households. A more detailed listing of food expenditures by individual product groups for the elderly households is available in Gallo et al. (1979).

The larger share of total expenditures used by the elderly for the purchase of food, health, and personal care products is of special significance in understanding the impact of price changes during the 1970s. Since food and medical prices increased faster than the overall rate of inflation during most of the 1970s, it is clear that the elderly were more directly affected by these relative price changes. On the other hand, transportation and housing are two other areas for which prices increased faster than the overall average. These changes did not have as much effect on the elderly given the budget proportions in Table 7.1. Decreases in prices of apparel and recreational activities relative to other commodities in recent years would not have had as much impact on the elderly relative to younger households in view of expenditure patterns.

Many of the differences in average expenditures and budget shares between the two age groups are consistent with general knowledge of how differences in household income and other factors influence expenditure behavior. For example, it is not surprising that health and personal care expenditures shown in Table 7.1 are positively related to age. Even though medical insurance of one form or another pays a high proportion of medical bills, it does not cover all bills for all individuals. Also, differences in expenditures for many of the categories are consistent with elderly households having lower incomes. The higher budget share for food associated with lower incomes can be viewed as empirical evidence of the low-income elasticity for food, thereby verifying Engel's Law that the proportion of income spent for food is higher among households with lower incomes. This is also consistent with the limited response in food expenditures by the elderly to changes in total expenditures estimated by Barnes and Zedlewski (1981). They also found expenditures on fuels and shelter (for renters) to be relatively unresponsive.

The only category in Table 7.1 for which expenditure behavior was not readily predictable from a priori knowledge about income and other factors was gifts and contributions. One reason this category may be bigger for older households, despite lower incomes, is that it may reflect the transfer of accumulated assets to younger generations. This interpretation is consistent with larger amounts of money which younger households report receiving as regular support contributions.

Although a number of tabulations of the Bureau of Labor Statistics data for several household characteristics are available in published form, the amount of information about expenditure patterns of the elderly is limited. Consequently, for further analyses, all observations for households with a head 55 years old or more were subjected to additional analyses. This group consisted of 3,629 and 3,576 households, respectively, in 1972 and 1973.

Expenditure Characteristics of the Elderly by Age

Total expenditures were substantially higher in 1973 than the previous year for each of the five subgroups of elderly households classified by age (see Table 7.2), but the relative magnitudes of the year-to-year differences were quite dissimilar, varying from 4.8 percent for the 75-and-older group to 21.6 percent for the 70–74 age group. The year-to-year differences in total expenditures were greater than the 6.2 percent increase in CPI for all except the oldest age group. These comparisons imply that in 1973 most of the elderly purchased a greater quantity of goods and services than in the previous year. Thus, their well-being was not adversely influenced by inflation. This is also consistent with the patterns of real incomes of the elderly, discussed in earlier chapters.

In order to compare differences for households of the same age cohort, the 1973 averages were recalculated based on respondents' age in 1972. For example, this permitted comparison of expenditures for households with heads who were 55 to 59 years of age in 1972 with those with heads 56 to 60 years of age in 1973. Tabulations for the other age subgroups in 1973 were modified in a similar manner in order to consider the same age cohorts over the two years. The results of these tabulations are reported in Table 7.3. Since this adjustment had no effect on the average for 1972, the 1972 values in Table 7.3 are the same as those in Table 7.2.

Comparing averages for the same age cohort instead of for similar age groups yielded smaller increases in expenditures between 1972 and 1973. For all groups, 1973 average expenditures exceeded 1972 levels, but the percentage increases were less than those indicated by the data in Table 7.2. Only in the 55–59 and 70–74 age cohorts was rate of change between 1972 and 1973 larger than the rate of inflation. Some of the differences could result from

TABLE 7.2. Average Expenditures by Age of Household Head for Those 55 Years of Age and Older, 1972–73 CES

Expenditure Category	Ages 55–59		Ages 60–64		Ages 65–69		Ages 70–74		Age 75 +	
	1972	1973	1972	1973	1972	1973	1972	1973	1972	1973
Food [a]	$1,969	$2,219	$1,657	$1,895	$1,385	$1,507	$1,108	$1,391	$1,023	$1,107
Housing	2,114	2,327	1,841	2,093	1,585	1,904	1,416	1,593	1,358	1,443
Apparel	628	663	464	554	353	409	279	311	197	205
Transportation	1,624	1,967	1,346	1,452	996	1,011	716	887	397	410
Health and personal care	662	717	631	677	541	604	498	599	491	504
Recreation	885	1,044	717	772	559	604	409	419	259	288
Insurance and pensions	813	972	581	733	257	283	135	218	104	84
Gifts and contributions	563	644	590	677	617	504	405	602	462	446
Taxes	2,076	2,398	1,617	1,787	745	969	300	385	301	324
Total expenditures	$11,334	$12,951	$9,444	$10,640	$7,038	$7,795	$5,266	$6,405	$4,592	$4,811

Source: Consumer Expenditure Survey, 1972–73 interviews.
[a] Includes alcohol and tobacco expenditures.

TABLE 7.3. Average Expenditures of Elderly Cohorts in 1972–73 CES

Expenditure Category	Ages 55–59 [a]		Ages 60–64 [a]		Ages 65–69 [a]		Ages 70–74 [a]		Age 75 + [a]	
	1972	1973	1972	1973	1972	1973	1972	1973	1972	1973
Food [b]	$1,969	$2,173	$1,657	$1,831	$1,385	$1,450	$1,108	$1,356	$1,023	$1,079
Housing	2,114	2,261	1,841	2,083	1,585	1,794	1,416	1,540	1,358	1,453
Apparel	628	639	464	525	353	372	279	292	197	203
Transportation	1,624	1,879	1,346	1,332	996	943	716	830	397	382
Health and personal care	662	717	631	665	541	591	498	582	491	503
Recreation	885	1,027	717	704	559	534	409	407	259	287
Insurance and pensions	813	962	581	610	257	240	135	206	104	82
Gifts and contributions	563	666	590	626	617	525	405	574	462	450
Taxes	2,076	2,320	1,617	1,541	745	852	300	375	301	328
Total expenditures	$11,334	$12,644	$9,444	$9,917	$7,038	$7,301	$5,266	$6,162	$4,592	$4,767

Source: Consumer Expenditure Survey, 1972–73 interviews.
[a] Age groups for 1973 were defined to include same age cohort as 1972.
[b] Includes alcohol and tobacco expenditures.

sample variability, but the latter two age cohorts definitely did not seem to be adversely affected by inflation between 1972 and 1973.

The differences in Tables 7.2 and 7.3 emphasize the difficulty of comparing changes in expenditures over time in order to identify the effects of inflation. If changes in expenditures for similar age groups over time, as presented in Table 7.2, are considered, some of the systematic differences due to life-cycle stages are eliminated. If data for specific age cohorts over time are considered as in Table 7.3, systematic changes in expenditures associated with aging are confounded with effects of inflation. In the latter case, however, it is possible to see changes in expenditure levels for the same group of people over time and to draw inferences about whether the real consumption levels have increased or decreased. A limitation of this type of inference, however, is that it is not possible to tell how much of the observed changes is the result of inflation without a separate estimate of the effects due to changing age. For every age cohort in Table 7.3, expenditures for food, housing, apparel, and health and personal care increased in absolute value between the two years. Some decreases were observed for each of the other categories. Decreases in expenditures for recreation were quite common. Only the youngest and oldest age cohorts reported increases in recreation expenditures between 1972 and 1973.

There was considerable similarity among the different age cohorts in the way total expenditures were allocated among different items. The share of total expenditures allocated to food, housing, and health and personal care tended to be larger for older households even though actual expenditures decreased. The proportion of total expenditures allocated to gifts and contributions also increased with age, even though actual amounts did not continuously increase with age. But these types of changes are not just an aging phenomenon, since income and average household size also vary with age, resulting in noticeable life-cycle expenditure patterns. Hamermesh (1982b) argues that declines in consumption as people age are the result of decisions to maximize lifetime satisfaction. This process assumes knowledge about the length of life but a high discounting of future periods' consumption. Deaton and Muellbauer (1980) also provide a detailed discussion of how various factors affect lifetime consumption patterns.

Increases in budget shares for food, housing, health and personal care were offset by declining proportions of total expenditures allocated to apparel, transportation, recreation, insurance and pension contributions, and taxes. These differences in budget allocation among age groups imply that changes in relative prices would not have the same effect on all elderly households. Higher prices of food, housing, and medical care not only would affect the elderly more than the rest of the population, but would also have an increasing impact with age among elderly households.

Total expenditures were a larger proportion of total income for the two youngest age cohorts in 1973 relative to 1972, but the three older age cohorts exhibited an opposite pattern of changes between 1972 and 1973. These values imply that the younger age groups may have decreased savings a little between 1972 and 1973. Groups in which retirement is more prevalent, however, may have increased savings some, although generally the rate of savings declines with age.

Differences by Marital Status and Race

Comparing expenditure patterns of elderly households classified by marital status indicated an increase of approximately $900 in expenditures for single females and married households between 1972 and 1973. The difference for single males was approximately $680. The relative rate of change for single households, however, was considerably larger than for married households. Increases in total expenditures were distributed among nearly all expenditure categories.

Within each year, married households had higher expenditures than single households in every category. Also, married households had a higher proportion of total expenditures allocated to transportation, recreation, insurance and pension contributions, and taxes relative to single elderly households. On the other hand, single households tended to spend larger proportions of their total expenditures for food and housing compared to married households. Among the two groups of single households, males spent more than females on food, transportation, recreation, taxes, and insurance and pension contributions. Categories for which single female households had higher expenditures were housing, apparel, and health and personal care.

A more detailed analysis of expenditures of married households indicated that differences between 1972 and 1973 were not the same for all age groups. Three of the five age groups were responsible for the increase in total expenditures of married households. A slight decrease in expenditures between 1972 and 1973 was reported for the 75-and-older age cohort. A somewhat larger decrease was also observed for the 65–69 age cohort. The difference for the latter group resulted from decreased expenditures for transportation, recreation, insurance and pension contributions, and gifts and contributions. For the 75-and-older group, the decrease resulted from smaller expenditures for food, housing, apparel, health and personal care, and insurance payments and pension contributions. In almost all other instances, increases in absolute levels of expenditure between 1972 and 1973 were observed. Food was the only category that showed a tendency to increase in relative importance between 1972 and 1973 for most age groups. This probably reflects food prices increasing between 1972 and 1973 at a faster rate than other commodities included in the CPI.

When CES households whose heads were 55 years of age or older in 1972 were classified by race, the change in total expenditure between the two years was in an opposite direction. Total expenditures by nonblacks were 11.6 percent higher in 1973 than in 1972, but for blacks there were expenditure declines. The distribution of expenditures among categories was very similar for the two years. In the case of blacks, food and housing, as well as gifts and contributions, increased in absolute and relative importance between 1972 and 1973. All other expenditure categories had absolute declines between the two years. It is difficult to know whether these differences reflect responses to inflation, other economic variables, or sample variability, since each year's data are for different groups of households.

Residence Differences

When households were classified by population density the largest year-to-year differences in expenditures were reported by the groups living outside a standard metropolitan statistical area (SMSA). The 21 percent increase in total expenditures for this group of households consisted of increases in all nine categories of expenditures.

The increases in total expenditures for households in metropolitan areas were much smaller. The change for those in medium and large SMSAs, however, was greater than the difference for the small-SMSA group. Inflation did not appear to decrease the real value of goods and services except for those in small SMSAs.

Despite the difference in total expenditures among the four residence groups, there was considerable similarity in the way the groups allocated their budgets each year. Nonmetropolitan households had higher budget shares for food, transportation, and health and personal care, but the shares of their budgets spent for apparel, recreation, and insurance and pensions were generally smaller than those of households in metropolitan areas.

Differences by Income Levels

To extend the examination of the effects of inflation and expenditure patterns at different income levels, the elderly component of the CES sample was divided into two subgroups. One subgroup of households consisted of those with annual incomes of $7,000 or less; the other group had incomes above $7,000. For the 1973 data, this classification resulted in 1,878 in the low-income category and 1,519 high-income households. The expenditures for each of these groups classified by age are presented in Table 7.4. The data indicate that lower-income households spent less for every category than higher-income households of the same age. Food, housing, and health and personal care, however, accounted for larger shares of total expenditures among lower-income households than among the higher-income subgroup. On the other hand, high-income households had substantially higher shares of total expenditures accounted for by insurance and pension, gifts and contributions, and taxes.

TABLE 7.4. Average Expenditures of High- and Low-Income Households for Those 56 Years of Age and Older in 1973

Expenditure Category	Ages 56-60		Ages 61-65		Ages 66-70		Ages 71-75		Age 76 +	
	Low	High	Low	High	Low	High	Low	High	Low	High
Food[a]	$1,528	$2,447	$1,397	$2,189	$1,201	$1,880	$1,126	$1,953	$ 931	$1,667
Housing	1,751	2,478	1,577	2,499	1,460	2,372	1,291	2,186	1,292	2,093
Apparel	433	727	311	701	253	577	192	552	157	385
Transportation	1,243	2,149	808	1,764	602	1,533	610	1,401	244	928
Health and personal care	559	785	498	802	460	817	459	902	418	842
Recreation	517	1,244	366	982	292	953	216	903	213	578
Insurance and pensions	320	1,235	194	952	105	472	75	549	42	238
Gifts and contributions	385	786	297	897	291	930	240	1,442	210	1,401
Taxes	281	3,188	170	2,668	87	2,177	52	1,213	39	1,476
Total expenditures	$7,017	$15,039	$5,618	$13,454	$4,751	$11,711	$4,261	$11,101	$3,546	$9,608

Source: Consumer Expenditure Survey, 1972–73 interviews.
Note: Low income is equivalent to $7,000 or less per year; high income is equivalent to greater than $7,000 annual income.
[a] Includes alcohol and tobacco expenditures.

An increasing proportion of the older age groups in the sample had lower incomes consistent with reduced labor force participation. For high-income as well as low-income households, however, total expenditures were negatively associated with age. This was also generally true for most individual categories, except in the case of health and personal care, and gifts and contributions for higher-income households. Expenditures for the latter two categories exhibited some increase with age among households with more than $7,000 annual income. These age-related differences are similar to those reported by Reinecke (1971) in his analysis of the 1960–61 Consumer Expenditure Survey. The contrast in the way in which health and personal care expenditures differed with age in the high- and low-income groups may reflect differences in the ability to purchase different amounts of services or the availability of subsidized medical services for the low-income elderly households. No information regarding the value of medical services provided by private or governmental insurance programs was available in this sample.

Differences in expenditure patterns for households that had marked differences in the proportion of expenditures allocated to the health and personal care category were also considered. For purposes of this analysis, households that spent less than 3 percent or more than 10 percent of their total budget for health and personal care in 1973 were identified for further study. This produced approximately 700 observations in each group. The high-medical-share households had absolute levels of health and personal care expenditures three to five times higher than those who had low shares of their total expenditures allocated to this category.

Households with high health and personal care expenditures had lower expenditures on every other category relative to comparable households that spent less than 3 percent of their budget on this item. Differences in the other categories more than offset the contrast in the health and personal care category resulting in smaller total expenditures. This pattern suggests that health impairments may have accounted for higher medical bills as well as for lower incomes. The extent to which the low-medical-share group consists of households with higher total expenditures may reflect higher levels of permanent income. Households with higher incomes throughout their lives may achieve improved health status through preventive health investments made at earlier ages, thereby reducing health expenditures during later stages of their life-cycle. The latter relationship would be consistent with explanations of inverse relationships between mortality and income reported by Cantrell (1982) and others.

Although all expenditure categories other than health and personal care were lower in absolute values in the presence of high medical bills, some of the largest differences were in the taxes, gifts, recreation, and transportation expenditure categories. Some of the differences in taxes undoubtedly resulted from a large fraction of medical expenditures being tax-deductible. Taxes would also be affected to the extent to which health impairments influence earning power. Among the more healthy and probably more affluent elderly, the proportion of total expenditures allocated to gifts and contributions increased quite significantly with age. There is no evidence of such a pattern among the households with high medical bills, which suggests that large and perhaps unexpected medical expenditures decrease discretionary income.

RHS EXPENDITURE PATTERNS

An alternative source of expenditure data for a selected age group of elderly households is the Retirement History Study (RHS). Information on food, housing, and some medical expenditure data consistently collected between 1969 and 1975 is available. We examined various components of these three categories of expenditures to see how they changed during this six-year period for the group of households included in the RHS. In particular, expenditures for food used at home and expenditures for food consumption away from home were considered. Three types of housing expenditures were available. One was a measure of home ownership expenditures, including mortgage, taxes, and property insurance payments; the other two categories consisted of the amount spent for rent and utilities. Two components of medical expenditures for which data were consistently available from the RHS over the entire six-year period were the amount spent for private medical insurance and the amount paid for hospital services. The medical expenditure categories do not represent the total value of medical services, but they constitute an important part of the total household medical bills not paid by insurance or other parties. One limitation of the medical data is that hospitalization costs refer only to the costs incurred when the respondent was hospitalized and do not necessarily reflect total household expenditures for hospital services. Information on private medical insurance premiums apparently includes the amount for the respondent as well as for the spouse. Chapter 8 focuses exclusively on medical expenditures and health status, extending the discussion in this chapter.

Examination of initial frequency distributions and summary statistics of expenditures identified a potential problem with some extremely large expenditure values. These were of concern because of their unusually large potential impact on the averages for particular subgroups in the sample. Consequently, the following upper limits were selected for the data used in preparing the following analysis: $250 per week for at-home food expenditures; $500 per week for away-from-home food expenditures; $40,000 per year for mortgage, taxes, and insurance; $20,000 per year for rent; $9,000 for utilities; $5,000 per year for private medical insurance premiums; and $20,000 per year for hospital costs paid by the respondent.

TABLE 7.5. Average Expenditures for Selected Items for Total RHS Sample, 1968–74

Expenditure Category	Actual Expenditures				Real Expenditures[a]			
	1968	1970	1972	1974	1968	1970	1972	1974
Food								
At home	$1,286	$1,302	$1,421	$1,592	$1,246	$1,168	$1,168	$ 980
Away from home	286	276	273	209	272	230	208	131
Housing								
Mortgage, taxes, insurance	526	568	579	585	506	478	455	388
Rent	267	243	250	261	247	205	194	173
Utilities	353	374	392	498	339	314	303	331
Medical								
Insurance premium	112	113	116	117	106	94	87	78
Hospital costs	20	19	23	19	19	15	17	13
Totals	$2,850	$2,895	$3,054	$3,281	$2,735	$2,504	$2,432	$2,094

Source: Retirement History Study, 1969–75 interviews.

[a] At-home and away-from-home food expenditures deflated by index of prices for at-home and away-from-home food components of CPI respectively. Housing and medical components deflated by housing and medical components of CPI, respectively.

Another difficulty with summarizing expenditure data from the RHS is that the values refer to different reference years. For example, expenditures for food were based on what respondents reported they "usually spent." Even though these data are supposedly representative of what was happening at the time of the survey, there may be substantial retrospective elements from the previous year influencing responses about usual expenditures. This information was combined with responses about housing and medical expenditures as well as income that specifically referred to the previous year. Thus, although the data were gathered in 1969, 1971, 1973, and 1975, the values are assumed to represent each of the previous years. Initially, average nominal expenditures for the entire sample of households from which data were available are reported. Comparisons also are made by deflating each of the categories by its respective components in the CPI.

Nominal and Real Expenditures for Entire Sample

The RHS data indicate sizable increases between 1968 and 1974 in total nominal expenditures on food, housing, and medical items (see Table 7.5). After adjusting for the effects of price increases, however, the real value of expenditures for these items declined by nearly $650 over the six years. The decrease in real expenditures was a little more than one-quarter of the decrease in real income, from $7,559 to $5,193 over the six-year period for this set of elderly households.

The data indicate that more income was spent on food, housing, and medical components in 1974 than 1968. Much of this change resulted from a larger proportion of income being spent on food at home and on utilities. The relative importance of home ownership costs increased some during the period, whereas expenditures for food away from home consistently decreased in relative importance. Food expenditure data in Table 7.5 are not identical to values reported by Murray (1978). Some of the differences can be attributed to the households included in the analyses. Murray used only households that provided data for multiple years and that reported food expenditures of $1 to $10,000 and incomes of $1 to $30,000. Our tabulations used all data except those exceeding the expenditure limits previously noted.

Actual expenditures on food at home tended to increase over the period. On the other hand, expenditures on food consumed away from home consistently declined, with a fairly substantial decline between 1972 and 1974. After the effects of price changes were removed, both types of food expenditures decreased between 1968 and 1974. In real terms, expenditures for food at home decreased by 21.4 percent. Some of this change can be explained by decreases in household size and real income as the respondents in this data base became progressively older. For example, average household size decreased by 11.8 percent between 1968 and 1974, which would be expected to decrease food consumption and expenditures by approximately the same proportion. The 31 percent decrease in real income would imply a 6.2 to 9.3 percent decrease in food expenditures, assuming an income elasticity of .2 or .3 for food. An estimate of .2 was reported by Murray (1978). Thus, the combined effects of the decreased household size and less real income would suggest an 18 to 21 percent decrease in at-home food expenditures. It is not too surprising that the relative decline in real value of purchases for food away from home was even bigger, since the income elasticity of demand for food away from home has generally been found to be larger than that for food at home. Estimates of the income elasticity for food away from home are provided by Prochaska and Schrimper (1973).

Some of the decrease in away-from-home expenditures between 1972 and 1974 might also be related to the increase in the price of gasoline and difficulties in obtaining it during this period. For the entire nation, however, away-from-home food expenditures increased in real terms during the same period, indicating that the gasoline shortage had little effect on eating away from home. The elderly may have been more responsive to the shortage than other age groups in the population.

Another effect that probably was contributing to the larger decrease in away-from-home expenditures for food is a tendency for households to substitute more food at home for away-from-home food as they become older. Some of this is undoubtedly in response to increased availability of time for food preparation as one or more members of the household leave the labor force. When one or more members of the household are working outside the home, they may find eating away from home to be especially convenient in conjunction with the location of their employment. This locational advantage of away-from-home dining dissipates with retirement. More evidence on this substitution at different stages of the life cycle is available in Fletcher (1981).

Expenditures for mortgage, taxes, insurance, and rent were consistently lower over time, after adjusting for the effects of price increases. Although nominal home ownership costs increased over the period, much of this is probably the result of increases in taxes and insurance, since it is likely that only a small proportion of the elderly would be assuming new mortgage payments. The extent to which some of the elderly were completing mortgage payments during the period would have a dampening effect on the overall averages for this item. After removing the effects of inflation, expenditures for utilities also decreased between 1968 and 1972, but they increased significantly between 1972 and 1974. In real terms, utility expenditures in 1974 were nearly the same as they were in 1968 for the elderly households included in the RHS.

Considerably less money was spent for private medical insurance premiums and hospital bills relative to food and housing expenditures. Hospital expenditures and medical insurance premiums showed little change in nominal terms over the six years. After removing the effects of higher prices of medical costs, the change in insurance premiums between 1968 and 1974 represented a decrease of 25 percent. The comparable decline in private costs for hospital care was more than 40 percent. Some of these changes can probably be attributed to the effect of medicare taking the place of private expenditures for some of the households as they became older.

Age Differences

The pattern of change in expenditures was quite similar for each of the age cohorts included in the sample. Between 1970 and 1974, the three two-year age groups had a 23 to 24 percent decline in real expenditures for food, housing, and the two medical components examined in this study (see Table 7.6). Expenditures were fairly similar in 1970 and 1972, but lower than the amounts reported in 1968. Changes between 1968 and 1970 as well as between 1972 and 1974 were fairly substantial for each group. As noted earlier, some of these changes over the four years are associated with decreases in average household size and real income as the respondents became older. Hamermesh (1982a) reports a slightly smaller rate of change in expenditures between the latter two years for a subsample of observations for which household size did not change. His measure is based on an estimate of total expenditures from information provided about selected categories in each year.

Expenditures for both types of food and home ownership generally decreased over time for each age group. Within each year, expenditures on these items tended to be inversely related to age. Hamermesh (1982a) also noted a tendency for total expenditures to decline with age among the elderly.

TABLE 7.6. Average Real Expenditures for Selected Items by 1968 Age Groups in RHS Sample, 1968–74

1968 Age and Expenditure category [a]	Average Expenditures			
	1968	1970	1972	1974
Age 57–58				
Food				
At home	$1,296	$1,211	$1,229	$1,024
Away from home	297	263	251	140
Housing				
Mortgage, taxes, insurance	590	546	522	350
Rent	237	194	187	157
Utilities	364	333	317	433
Medical				
Insurance premium	108	99	114	93
Hospital costs	20	13	23	16
Totals	$2,912	$2,659	$2,643	$2,215
Age 59–60				
Food				
At home	$1,264	$1,163	$1,162	$ 986
Away from home	265	234	189	116
Housing				
Mortgage, taxes, insurance	497	489	439	369
Rent	237	207	183	160
Utilities	334	306	301	327
Medical				
Insurance premium	99	96	84	72
Hospital costs	15	15	20	11
Totals	$2,711	$2,511	$2,378	$2,041
Age 61–62				
Food				
At home	$1,175	$1,128	$1,109	$ 926
Away from home	252	192	181	137
Housing				
Mortgage, taxes, insurance	415	385	390	232
Rent	269	214	212	187
Utilities	312	300	290	310
Medical				
Insurance premium	110	66	62	67
Hospital costs	15	15	20	11
Totals	$2,549	$2,300	$2,263	$1,961

Source: Retirement History Study, 1969–75 interviews.
Note: At-home and away-from-home expenditures deflated by index of prices for at-home and away-from-home food components of CPI respectively. Housing and medical components deflated by housing and medical components of CPI, respectively.
[a] Age of respondent in 1968.

The same pattern was observed for utility expenditures until 1974, when general increases for each of the age groups occurred. Real rent expenditures tended to decrease over time but generally were positively related to age. There was some tendency for health insurance premiums and private hospital costs to decrease over time and with age, but the changes were not as systematic as other expenditure components examined. These decreases are not too surprising in view of the effects of medicare benefits noted earlier.

Comparisons can also be made across years for different age groups to see the effect of inflation on real expenditures net of age effects. For example, the 1970 expenditures for the first age group can be compared to corresponding values reported by the 59–60 age group in 1968. Similarly, the 1972 expenditures for the 57–58 age cohort can be compared with the 1970 expenditures for the 59–60 age group and the 1968 expenditures for the 61–62 age group. If it is assumed that in the absence of inflation year-to-year changes for a given age cohort would have been like the differences between age groups in previous years, the net effect of inflation can be observed. In other words, this amounts to anticipating the same changes over time for a given cohort as those observed among different age groups at a given point in time.

A comparison of total expenditures at a given age across the three cohorts indicates more similarity than is evident by looking at differences in any row or column in Table 7.6. In two of three cases the youngest age cohort indicated a decrease from corresponding values for the 59–60 age group in the preceding period. Similarly, in two of the three years the second oldest cohort also had a decrease in expenditures from corresponding values of the older age group in the preceding period. In each instance between 1970 and 1972, real expenditures increased somewhat. However, decreases in real expenditures occurred between 1968 and 1970 and again between 1972 and 1974.

Differences by Other Household Characteristics

When the sample was classified by marital status, decreases in real expenditures were observed for each group. Changes in total expenditures over the six years were slightly smaller for single males and females than for couples. This probably results from real incomes of singles declining less than that of couples over the period. Nevertheless, single males and females spent much more of their income for the selected categories than couples.

At-home food expenditures generally decreased more for couples than for single males or females. In fact, the two single groups had an increase between 1968 and 1970. Single males had the largest expenditures for food away from home and the lowest medical insurance expenditures in each period. Over time their away-from-home food expenditures changed in a manner similar to the pattern for couples and single females, accounting for a substantial decrease in the proportion of their income. For all groups, medical insurance expenditures changed in about the same proportion as incomes. Singles spent more on rents and less on home ownership than couples, which is consistent with differences in home ownership among marital groups.

For each race, changes in real expenditures over the four survey years were very similar. Thus, the changes observed in the aggregate RHS sample appeared to be experienced by each race. Expenditures on selected items, however, accounted for markedly different proportions of real income for the two races. Food, housing, and the two medical components accounted for considerably larger shares of real income for nonwhite households than for white households. In nearly every instance, expenditures reported by whites exceeded expenditures reported by nonwhites.

When the sample was classified by urbanization characteristics, very similar changes in total expenditures were observed over the six years for each group of households. Respondents in areas with more than 250,000 population consistently had the highest expenditures for food, rent, and home ownership. Utility expenditures were consistently smaller in the large urban areas than in either of the other two urbanization categories considered. Nonurbanized residents paid the most for private medical insurance premiums in three of the four years. No systematic differences were observed between hospital costs and urbanization.

The differences in total expenditures across the urbanization categories were consistent with differences in average incomes. Consequently, fairly similar proportions of income were spent on the selected items among different urbanizations within each year. There was a tendency for these proportions to increase over time as a result of the decreases in real incomes exceeding expenditure adjustments. This was especially true for food at home and for utilities.

Our analysis of expenditure data for elderly households in the 1972–73 Consumer Expenditure Survey and from the 1969–75 part of the Retirement History Study indicates substantial differences among various subgroups over time. The CES data suggest that most of the elderly increased expenditures proportionately more than the rate of change in prices. The comparisons also imply that the experiences of particular age cohorts differ from that for particular age groups. Different budget allocations among age groups indicate that changes in relative prices have different impacts on segments of the elderly population. Higher prices of food and medical care not only affect the elderly more than the rest of the population, but also have an increasing impact with age on the elderly population.

The decrease in real expenditures for selected food, housing, and medical items between 1968 and 1974 in the Retirement History Study was not as large as the decrease in real income. After controlling for age effects, the analysis suggested that inflation may have been associated with a decrease in real expenditures for elderly households for the above items between 1968 and 1970 and again between 1972 and 1974. However, the level of real expenditures appeared to increase between 1970 and 1972, implying a mixed effect of inflation on well-being. Of course, these changes in expenditures also reflect responses to declines in real income for other reasons.

8 Personal Health Expenditures and Well-being in the Later Years

THE PROBLEM

Personal expenditures for health care among adults increase with age, and societal expenditures for health care in the United States have increased dramatically in recent decades as the population has aged. Epidemiological research has documented that in adulthood the risk of chronic disease and functional impairment increases with age. As is the case of all generalizations about older adults, however, epidemiological evidence documents substantial variation in the incidence and prevalence of chronic disease among older adults, particularly differences between relatively younger and older elderly, between males and females, and between older adults of higher and lower socioeconomic status. Further, social-scientific research has documented increased demand for and utilization of health care by older individuals and the economic cost of that care. Personal and public expenditures for health care tend to be about three times higher for older adults than for adults generally. The proportion of the gross national product devoted to health care in the United States, and in industrial societies generally, is now above 10 percent and growing; the cost of geriatric care contributes significantly to the observed cost. Inflation of health care services costs in recent decades has been increasing at a rate considerably above the rate for other goods and services (see, e.g., Shanas and Maddox, 1976; Wan, 1982; Maddox, 1981; Hickey, 1980; Fries, 1981; Roos and Shapiro, 1981; and Andersen et al., 1975).

Research on the utilization of health care services by older adults indicates that older adults are more likely to consume such services than are younger persons. A minority of older adults demand more services than their objective health status appears to warrant (they have been called "the worried well"), and another minority demands less care than an experienced clinician would expect ("the deniers"). But, on average, the great majority of older consumers of health care services appear to be realistic in their demand for services (Haug, 1981; Andersen et al., 1975). There are, however, several important aspects about the consumption of health care services in the later years that are less well documented and understood. For example:

1. The incidence and prevalence of chronic conditions are known to increase with age among adults, but the differential distribution of functional

impairments related to these chronic conditions among older adults has not been adequately documented. The differential risk of pathology that produces functional impairment with increasing age among identified subgroups of older adults (e.g., the old vs. the very old; males vs. females; economically secure vs. poverty-level income) has not been as adequately documented as for adult populations generally. References to the health status or health care utilization of *the elderly* are increasingly suspect.

2. Differential personal (out-of-pocket) expenditures for the purchase of health care, changes in their expenditures over time, and the ratio of out-of-pocket expenditures to the total cost of personal health care have not been adequately documented. This is especially the case for subgroups of older adults with different sociodemographic and health characteristics (gender, economic status, education, functional status).

3. Particularly scarce is evidence about the demand for health care in response to expected age-related deterioration in functional status (well-being), the declining financial status of older consumers, and the rising costs of health care. These three factors — occasions for seeking health care, declining financial status, and inflating cost — would necessarily interact in affecting demand for care. But the effect is not obvious. The occasions for care increase with age, but the decreased economic capacity to purchase care and cost inflation are potentially offsetting. We know very little about the income and price elasticity of the demand for health care generally, and even less about the elasticity of demand by older adults.

4. The first three aspects focus on descriptions of differential functional capacity among older adults and differences in personal expenditures for health care as they age. A fourth aspect concentrates on the explication of observed behavior in the purchase of health care among older adults and the health consequences of that behavior. Two theoretical questions of particular importance emerge. One is concerned with understanding elasticity of demand for health care in the later years and possible age-related changes in perceived (subjective) utility of such investments. The second concentrates on the objective consequences of differential personal investment in health care for the well-being of older adults. Two competing theoretical perspectives might explain how older consumers who, on average, experience declining functional capacity might behave in purchasing health care.

One theoretical perspective that emphasizes health care as an item of consumption suggests that older consumers, like health professionals, assign top priority to health as a value, perceive investment in health care as likely to produce an improvement in functional status (or at least to ameliorate decline), and reflect that perceived utility of investing in health care in their consumer expenditures which increases with age as functional capacity declines. An alternative perspective, suggested by human capital theory (Grossman, 1972; Menefee, 1980; see also Newhouse and Phelps, 1973), proposes a different explanation and prediction. This perspective, which emphasizes health care as an investment in human capital, suggests that older adults develop a realistic expectation of decline in functional capacity with age by both older individuals and health care providers, a decline that increased investment in health care is perceived as unlikely to be able to reverse. Consequently, on average, neither a rational older consumer nor a health care provider attempts to offset decline in functioning completely by increased investment in health care. Put another way, older adults and health care providers have increasingly modest expectations about the ability of health care to ensure functional capacity and restrict their investment in health care accordingly.

These alternative perspectives have very different implications for explaining and predicting the elasticity of demand for health care among older adults and the objective consequences of differential investment in health with age. The first perspective suggests that, although the older consumer and providers expecting functional decline might attempt to increase investment in health, increased cost of care might decrease the demand for health care and that the likely outcome of this decreased demand is an increase in functional incapacity. Unlimited increase in health care as needed is, in this view, desirable but constrained by economic resources. The alternative perspective suggests in contrast that, although inflation of health care cost may decrease demand for health care, other factors contribute to an expected decrease in the purchase of health care with age. Specifically, the decrease in demand for health care may reflect a subjective but rational assessment of the lowered utility of personal consumption of health care in the later years on the part of both older individuals and health care providers. If this is the case, an observed age-related reduction in consumption of health care would reflect reduced perceived utility of formal health care. Inflation in health care costs might augment the tendency to reduce the purchase of care with age but would not explain the decrease. There is, in fact, some evidence that highly technical, high-cost medical care may have limited utility in reducing functional incapacity or in effecting rehabilitation of chronic illness (Enthoven, 1980). While we have only limited evidence that older consumers or providers consider such information subjectively in making decisions about the care prescribed or purchased, a perspective that considers health care as an investment calls attention to the possibility that perceived efficacy is a relevant consideration.

METHOD

The data used in the analysis are from the Retirement History Study (RHS) of the Social Security Administration, and specifically from observations made in the first three rounds of observations of that survey in 1969,

1971, and 1973 (Maddox, Fillenbaum, and George, 1979; Motley, 1975; Wan, 1982). It was not feasible to use the 1975 data in this analysis, since the type of medical expenditure data collected was more limited for that year than for the earlier years. Observation of the RHS panel over a period of four years, however, provides a rare opportunity to assess longitudinal trends in health and in health care expenditures. Observed changes over time reflect, in part, the aging of panelists, but more than aging is involved. Among panelists of the same age, gender and socioeconomic status affect health and health care expenditures. Further, while a formal cohort analysis was not undertaken, differences among age-cohorts in the panel are suggested by the evidence reviewed.

Assessing Functional Capacity

Our measurement of functional capacity follows a procedure developed by Fillenbaum (Fillenbaum and Landerman, 1981) which dichotomizes functional capacity as unimpaired or impaired on three dimensions – physical health, subjective well-being (a proxy for mental health status), and capacity for self-care. Measurement of functional status for these three dimensions was derived from a widely used multidimensional assessment strategy developed at Duke University (Duke Center, 1978; Maddox, 1981). The Retirement History Study was not designed originally to include the Duke functional assessment procedures, but the study did collect data amenable to the construction of comparable scales. Summary classifications of functioning as impaired or unimpaired for the dimensions of physical health, subjective well-being, and capacity for self-care reasonably approximating the original Duke classifications were derived.

The Retirement History Study began in 1969 with a probability sample of 11,153 men and nonmarried women aged 58–63. The intention was to treat the sample as a panel to be interviewed at intervals of two years over a decade in which subjects would move from the work force into retirement (Motley, 1975). The interview schedule provided relatively detailed information about economic variables. Maddox, Fillenbaum, and George (1979) demonstrated that a variety of questions on the interview schedule could be used to develop measures of functional status (health, mental health, and self-care capacity) analogous to those developed in studies of normal aging at Duke University. Factor analysis was used to identify groups within twenty-eight questions in the RHS interview which cohered around concepts of physical health, subjective well-being, and capacity for self-care. A stratified random sample ($N = 599$) was used in this analysis. Further, another stratified random sample ($N = 277$) was used to determine that machine scoring of subjects as impaired or unimpaired on the three relevant dimensions of functioning agreed with experienced raters working from data in the interview protocols. The level of agreement between the ratings of experienced reviewers and those of the machine was very high (physical functioning, 93 percent; subjective well-being, 100 percent; capacity for self-care, 98 percent).

The intercorrelations between the three dimensions of the index of functional impairment (IFI) used in this chapter found in a subsample of 599 were as follows: physical functioning/subjective well-being, 0.40; subjective well-being/capacity for self care, 0.28; and physical functioning/capacity for self-care, 0.83. Although the last of these correlations is relatively high ($R^2 = 0.64$) and reflects the artifact of overlapping questions in the two dimensions, this component was retained because it added an increment of special relevance in identifying a high level of functional impairment.

The pattern of intercorrelations of the dichotomized components of each of the three dimensions used to construct the index of functional incapacity was similar to that reported above, though the correlations were consistent but slightly lower in each instance.

Six types of RHS information were used to assess *physical health status* — self-assessment of health, reported health problems, handicaps, disabilities, work limitations, and work capacity. Three questions were used to classify subjects in terms of *subjective well-being* — a question about happiness, a question about satisfaction with living situation, and a question about how the subject perceived his or her well-being compared with that of peers. Eight questions were used to assess the *capacity for self-care* in daily activities; six of the questions overlapped with items used to assess physical health but were scored to identify individuals indicating severe limitations such as being confined to bed, inability to leave home, and inability to use public transportation. This activities of daily living (ADL) indicator is not a precise analog of the Duke Older Americans Resources and Services (OARS) ADL scale but is a reasonable indicator of individuals at highest risk for dependence on others for care. The details of the questions used for classification of subjects on the three dimensions of physical, behavioral, and self-care functional capacity and scoring procedures are presented in Fillenbaum and Landerman (1981). For the analysis of data presented below, an index of functional impairment summarizes the three dichotomized dimensions of functioning; the index ranges from 0 (no functional impairment on any of the three dimensions) to 3 (functional impairment on all three dimensions).

Health Expenditures and Economic Classification

Health expenditures of two types are documented: (1) annual out-of-pocket expenditures and (2) total annual health bills. The reported out-of-pocket and total expenditures that constitute personal consumption or investments in health either as preventive health maintenance or as an investment intended to contain the effects of illness are summed for each year. Admittedly we cannot determine directly from the data available in the Retirement

History Study the subjective intentions of the health care expenditures reported, and at best we can only make inferences about possible intentions from reported behavior and outcomes. The data include detailed reports on annual health insurance payments and the personal cost of hospitalization, doctor's charges, prescription drugs, and other health care expenses. Personal health care expenditures, when related to the total cash income from all sources reported for the family unit, constitute the *health share* of the subject's budget. Total health bills include literally *all* charges for medical, hospital, and related care whether these bills were paid by insurance, by an employer, or by others. The exact wording of the questions that produced the answers from which annual expenditure estimates are made is found in Motley (1975). It should be noted that in each survey year (1969, 1971, 1973), the report of annual expenditures is for the prior year. Although definitive confirmation of the reliability and validity of self-reported out-of-pocket and total health care expenditures is not possible, available evidence indicates that the levels of accuracy are acceptable.

The reliability and validity of self-reported out-of-pocket and total health care expenditures in survey research are relatively recent interests. Definitive research on these issues does not exist, but Marquis (1980) summarizes relevant recent research and concludes that the best available evidence reveals no systematic response bias in self-reported health care expenditures when these expenditures are checked with objectively recorded expenditures. Specifically, no systematic bias in self-reporting has been found for either total or out-of-pocket expenditures. The bias that does exist appears to be relatively small (i.e., less than 10 percent error), not statistically significant, and random, and hence offsetting.

Since functional impairment and health expenditures are both known to be related to economic status, for purposes of analysis subjects were dichotomized as being economically unimpaired or impaired, using as a point of reference federal guidelines for an intermediate budget for workers in 1969, 1971, and 1973. Although most subjects were employed at the initial observation in 1969, a minority did retire over the next four years included in the observations. For retirees, therefore, the procedure used tends to overstate economic impairment. In any case, the classification of a subject as economically unimpaired if total cash income was at least 82 percent of the federal guidelines for intermediate budget for workers appears to be reasonable (Fillenbaum and Landerman, 1981). Although an individual's economic status can and did change over time, individuals with the same status at all three observations are identified in the tables that follow.

Our descriptive analysis reports summary measures of trends in functional status and personal expenditures over three periods of observation both for the total sample and for different sociodemographic subgroups. Distinctions by gender proved to be particularly important in the analysis, as did both economic status and functional capacity status. Further, we note two potentially significant changes that occurred during the period under consideration. First, an increasing percentage of the sample retired and hence experienced a reduction in earned income. Second, an increasing percentage of the sample was eligible for medicare or could rely on medicaid, which became fully operational after 1970.

Our explanatory analysis concentrated on the behavior and experience over time of significant or critical subgroups in the total population. For example, a critical subgroup was composed of individuals who at the first observation and both subsequent observations were functionally unimpaired, economically unimpaired, and relatively well educated. This subgroup illustrates older adults whose behavior illustrates personal expenditures in health under conditions most likely to reflect an optional investment in human capital. In contrast, there is the subgroup which at all three observations was impaired in terms of functional capacity and economic status and had less than a high school education. This subgroup represents individuals subjected to a maximum functional impairment and minimum resources for responding. A comparison of these groups provides some insight into elasticity of health care expenditures under extreme differences in income. Intermediate to these subgroups are those that initially have unimpaired functional status but are challenged at subsequent observations by health events requiring hospitalization. Their personal expenditures for health in the period subsequent to this challenge warrant study regarding possible change in health investment strategy.

For all the subgroups of interest the general question posed is: Does the observed differential investment in health reflected in personal investment in health care modify the general tendency toward reduced functional capacity over time typically experienced by older persons in the study population?

FINDINGS

Functional Status

Functional status, defined as the number of impaired dimensions out of the possible three (physical health, subjective well-being, and capacity for self-care), tended, as expected, to decline over time in this population of older adults. About 50 percent of RHS subjects at the first observation were unimpaired on all three functional dimensions; this is consistent with findings of other surveys using similar measures of functional impairment (e.g., Maddox, 1981). Our analysis indicates that no one of the three components of our composite index of functional status contributed disproportionately to the summary score. On average, the summary index of functional impairment (IFI), which was 0.82 in 1969, increased to 0.92 in 1971 and to 1.12 in 1973

TABLE 8.1. Index of Functional Impairment of RHS Respondents, 1969-73

	Year (Mean and Standard Deviation)			Average Annual Difference in Index Mean	% Change 1969 to 1973
Subjects	1969	1971	1973		
Total sample	0.82	0.92	1.12	0.15	36.6
$N = 8,928$	(1.04)	(1.08)	(1.13)		
Males	0.79	0.87	1.11	0.16	40.5
$N = 6,414$	(1.00)	(1.05)	(1.13)		
Females	1.05	1.06	1.16	0.055	10.5
$N = 2,514$	(1.12)	(1.13)	(1.14)		
Economically unimpaired					
(all 3 observations)	0.40	0.43	0.65	0.125	62.5
$N = 3,272$	(0.70)	(0.74)	(0.91)		
Economically impaired					
(all 3 observations)	1.53	1.56	1.66	0.065	8.5
$N = 2,766$	(1.45)	(1.16)	(1.13)		
Educational Attainment					
11 years or less	1.04	1.11	1.31	0.135	26.0
$N = 5,430$	(1.09)	(1.12)	(1.15)		
12-15 years	0.64	0.70	0.89	0.125	39.0
$N = 2,728$	(0.92)	(0.97)	(1.06)		
16 or more years	0.38	0.42	0.59	0.105	55.3
$N = 770$	(0.74)	(0.75)	(0.89)		

Source: Retirement History Study, 1969-73 interviews.
Note: The number of subjects in this analysis is less than the total number of subjects in the total initial sample of 1969 because we included only subjects on whom relevant information was available in the first three rounds of the study (1969, 1971, and 1973). In the RHS, the health status data and other personal characteristics are for the interview years, that is, 1969, 1971, and 1973. The income and expenditure data reported in Tables 8.2, 8.3, 8.4, 8.5, and 8.6 are for years just prior to the interview, that is, 1968, 1970, and 1972.

(see Table 8.1). The IFI increased about 12 percent in the two years between observations from 1969 to 1971 and 22 percent from 1971 to 1973. In general, this increasing impairment holds for all sociodemographic subgroups in the study population, although the consistently high standard deviations and the higher initial IFI but smaller increase in the index for females should be noted. Those subgroups with the highest initial index of impairment in 1969 (females, impaired income, less education) had lower rates of decline over the next two observations. Also, the female/male ratio of the index in 1969 was 1.33 and in 1973 was 1.04. The ratio of the index of the economically impaired compared with the economically unimpaired for 1969 was 3.83 and in 1973 was 2.55. The ratio of the index for the least and most educated in 1969 was 2.74 and in 1973 was 2.22. Although the differentiation among subgroups in impairment tends to decline in every instance, the initial ranking is maintained.

Beyond the consistently increasing functional decline with age across subgroups and the substantial within-group variance, two additional observations from analyses not shown are notable. First, there is no evidence of age-cohort differences in the trajectory of functional decline among RHS subjects. Cross-sectionally in 1969, there is a consistent increase in functional impairment for subjects in each year of age, 58 to 63. This pattern is repeated in 1971 (when subjects were 60 to 65) and 1973 (when subjects were 62 to 67). For each specific age, the ratio of the index of functional impairment for an age group in 1969 compared with the index of the same group in 1973 is essentially the same, ranging between 0.76 and 0.78.

Second, although increase in functional impairment is a function of age, the observed variance is a reminder that the aging process is complex. Individuals observed to be functionally unimpaired or very impaired in 1969 had a high probability of remaining unimpaired or very impaired in 1971 and 1973. This was the case for about 66 percent of the unimpaired and 60 percent of the very impaired. However, individuals with intermediate levels of impairment initially (one or two functional dimensions impaired) displayed considerable variability in the direction of movement on the index of impairment. As many as 60 percent of subjects in the middle range showed either improved or worsened conditions in both 1971 and 1973 as compared to their functional status in 1969.

Investment in Health Care

Expenditures reported in 1969, 1971, and 1973 indicate a trend of decreased investment in health for the years 1968, 1970, and 1972. This trend, with the exception of subjects who have at least a college education, holds for all sociodemographic subgroups (see Table 8.2). Declining personal (out-of-pocket) health expenditures is unexpected, given the observed trajectory of functional impairment (see Table 8.1). The mean out-of-pocket expenditures for the total sample and by sex in 1968 are very similar to the estimates of the National Center for Health Statistics reported for 1970. The means for the RHS sample in 1970 of $249 for the total sample and $196 for females and $267 for males have as their corresponding figures reported by the National Center for Health Statistics in 1970, the amounts of $257, $245, and $261.

Again, differentiation among subgroups and stability of the ranking of the subgroups over time should be noted. The male/female ratio of mean expenditures was 1.32 in 1968 and remained 1.30 in 1972. The ratio of economically unimpaired to economically impaired was 1.56 in 1968 and 1.90 in 1972. The ratio of the highest to lowest in education was 1.57 in 1968 and 1.86 in 1972.

We now turn to the estimate of health shares in the budgets of the study population (Table 8.3). In this analysis we have removed a small number of subjects who report personal health expenditures considerably above reported total cash income. The data indicate relative stability of the health share over the three observations. The average health share of the sample is in

TABLE 8.2. Mean Personal Health Expenditures of RHS Respondents, 1968–72, in Constant Dollars (1967 = 100)

Subjects	Year			% Change 1969 to 1972
	1968	1970	1972	
Total sample N = 8,928	$247	$249	$218	− 11.7
Females N = 2,514	$201	$196	$179	− 10.9
Males N = 6,414	265	267	233	− 12.1
Economically unimpaired (all 3 observations) N = 3,272	284	296	266	− 6.3
Economically impaired (all 3 observations) N = 2,766	182	158	140	− 23.0
Educational Attainment				
11 years or less N = 5,430	217	216	185	− 14.7
12–15 years N = 2,728	283	283	247	− 12.7
16 or more years N = 770	341	360	344	+ 0.8

Source: Retirement History Study, 1969–73 interviews.

Note: Personal health expenditures include health insurance premiums, hospital care, doctor visits and treatment, prescription drugs, and other services and supplies (nursing care, physical therapy, hearing aids, etc.).

the range frequently estimated in the literature (about 6 percent). But again the differences by subgroups are substantial. In general, those subgroups noted previously to have the worst functional impairment status (i.e., females, the economically impaired, and the least educated) report health shares of about 10 percent. In 1968, for example, the female/male ratio for health shares was 2.00; the economically impaired/unimpaired ratio was 2.9; and the ratio of least/highest educational attainment was 1.66. Although slightly reduced, these ratios remain relatively high and in the same direction in 1972. It should be noted further that those subgroups with the highest shares nonetheless spent fewer dollars for health care (see Table 8.2). For example, in 1968 females whose average share of income allocated to health was 10 percent reported personal expenditures of $201. In contrast, males whose health share was 5 percent reported out-of-pocket expenditures of $265. Finally, for the total sample and for each subgroup the share of income spent for health care remained relatively constant over a period of four years. The exceptions are the subgroups with the greatest economic security and the most education. The increase in budget shares observed in the subgroups between 1968 and 1972 moved them toward but left them below the average

TABLE 8.3. Health Share of Total Personal Income of RHS Respondents, 1968–72 (Percent)

Subjects	Year			% Change 1968 to 1972
	1968	1970	1972	
Total sample	6.0	7.0	7.0	16.7
	(N = 8,190)	(N = 7,950)	(N = 7,896)	
Females	10.0	9.8	9.8	– 2.0
	(N = 2,154)	(N = 2,003)	(N = 2,054)	
Males	5.0	5.8	6.1	22.0
	(N = 6,036)	(N = 5,947)	(N = 5,842)	
Economically unimpaired (all 3 observations) N = 3,224	3.5	4.1	4.3	22.9
Economically impaired (all 3 observations) N = 2,402	10.0	9.9	9.6	– 4.0
Educational attainment (all 3 observations)				
11 years or less N = 4,970	6.8	7.1	7.4	8.9
12–15 years N = 2,728	6.1	6.7	6.7	9.8
16 or more years N = 770	4.1	4.9	5.8	41.5

Source: Retirement History Study, 1969–73 interviews.

budget share of the total sample in 1972. The next highest percentage increase observed was among the economically unimpaired whose share increased from .035 to .043. The percentage change in health share is relatively large over the period of observation, but the greatest change is found where the initial share is smallest.

The pattern of personal investment in health as reflected in health shares over time by subjects of different ages is notable. In an analysis not shown, the oldest subjects in the study — those 63 years of age initially — tended to invest a relatively constant share of total cash income in health (about 7.6 percent) in 1968, 1970, and 1972. Subjects at each age included in the sample display a tendency to move toward this percentage over the four years observed. The ratio of the health share investment for each chronological age group in 1968 compared with the health share of the oldest group in 1970 moves from 0.77 at age 58 continuously to 1.00 at ages 62 and 63. Similarly, the ratio of the health shares of those aged 58 to those aged 63 in 1968 is 0.70, and by 1972 the ratio is 0.91. In sum, the health share appears to peak and hold between the range of 7 to 8 percent at about age 63. As will be indicated below, the observed pattern apparently is not an artifact of the availability of insurance or payment of health bills by others.

TABLE 8.4. Personal Expenditures for Medical Services of RHS Respondents in 1968 and 1972 (1967 Dollars)

Expenditures for Medical Services in 1968	Total	Insured	Not Insured	Economi- cally Unimpaired	Economi- cally Impaired
Number reporting	8,100	6,373	1,697	4,438	3,590
Median					
All reporting	$ 58	$ 71	$ 24	$ 71	$ 47
Reporting $1 or more	94	99	63	97	86
Mean					
All reporting	$157	$167	$126	$166	$148
Reporting $1 or more	201	206	182	203	200
Mean ratio of expenditures to bills for those with bills of $1 or more in 1968	.86	.86	.89	.86	.87

Expenditures for Medical Services in 1972	Total	Insured	Not Insured	Economi- cally Unimpaired	Economi- cally Impaired
Number reporting	8,059	7,142	917	4,088	3,848
Median					
All reporting	$ 60	$ 66	$ 23	$ 75	$ 45
Reporting $1 or more	91	91	62	98	78
Mean					
All reporting	$143	$148	$108	$158	$127
Reporting $1 or more	176	178	154	186	164
Mean ratio of expenditures to bills for those with bills of $1 or more in 1972	.83	.82	.89	.82	.83

Source: Retirement History Study, 1969–73 interviews.

Note: Medical services include hospital care, doctor visits and treatments, prescription drugs, and other services and supplies (nursing care, physical therapy, hearing aids, etc.) but not health insurance payments.

The availability of health insurance or equivalent public payment for health care is associated with increased health expenditures (National Center for Health Services Research, 1977; Andersen et al., 1975). In 1968 almost all subjects in the RHS study population (unless disabled) were too young to be eligible for medicare, and medicaid was not fully activated as a federal program until after 1970. By the third round of the RHS study in 1973, most subjects were eligible for medicare, and medicaid was operational. An analysis of reported personal expenditures and total annual expenditures for health care comparing 1968 and 1972 is useful. Personal (out-of-pocket) expenditures for these two years are reported in Table 8.4 (above) with health insurance premium payments removed. The previously observed pattern (see Table 8.2) of declining personal investment in health care is generally repeated, particularly in the most relevant comparisons of mean expenditures among those who reported the purchase of some health services. Significantly, reduced

TABLE 8.5. Bills for Medical Services of RHS Respondents in 1968 and 1972 (1967 Dollars)

Bills for Medical Services in 1968	Total	Insured	Not Insured	Economically Unimpaired	Economically Impaired
Number reporting	7,738	6,175	1,532	4,320	3,351
Median					
All reporting	$ 71	$ 80	$ 38	$ 80	$ 57
Reporting $1 or more	114	118	94	118	113
Mean					
All reporting	$251	$271	$173	$277	$220
Reporting $1 or more	324	337	262	340	303

Bills for Medical Services in 1972	Total	Insured	Not Insured	Economically Unimpaired	Economically Impaired
Number reporting	7,392	6,569	823	3,805	3,475
Median					
All reporting	$ 75	$ 82	$ 36	$ 94	$ 58
Reporting $1 or more	115	119	94	128	105
Mean					
All reporting	$268	$282	$158	$301	$232
Reporting $1 or more	336	346	238	357	310

Source: Retirement History Study, 1969–73 interviews.

Note: Medical services include hospital care, doctor visits and treatments, prescription drugs, and other services and supplies (nursing care, physical therapy, hearing aids, etc.) but not health insurance payments.

out-of-pocket expenditures are observed among the insured (78 percent of the subjects in this analysis) as well as the uninsured and among the economically unimpaired as well as the economically impaired. Note also that the percentage of total expenditures accounted for by out-of-pocket payments is slightly reduced in 1972 but still remains high (more than 80 percent).

The declining out-of-pocket expenditures shown in Table 8.4 coupled with the relatively constant proportion of personal expenditures to total bills for health care anticipates the data on medical bills (total expenditures) summarized in Table 8.5. Total expenditures in constant dollars increased only slightly (4 percent) from 1968 to 1972 for the study population and even less for the insured (80 percent of subjects in the analysis). Total expenditures for the uninsured decreased 9 percent during this period.

DETERMINANTS OF DEMAND FOR HEALTH CARE

A review of the evidence of general decline in functional capacity with age (Table 8.1), matched with a declining constant dollar personal investment in health care and a relatively stable share of income spent on health care

(Tables 8.2 and 8.3), suggests variation in the demand for health care in relation, variously, to functional status, income, and the cost of health care.
Since the ratio of out-of-pocket expenditures to total reported health expenditures on average declined only slightly during the period under study, this
means that study subjects tended on average to spend less on health care
between 1968 and 1972.

Holtzmann and Olsen (1978), in a comprehensive review of relevant conceptual issues and evidence on elasticity in the personal demand for health
care, conclude that the quantity of care purchased is affected relatively less by
the price of care and the waiting time required to secure care and relatively
more by income. They note further that a precise analysis of price and income
elasticity in the demand for health care is affected substantially by the
availability of health insurance. Finally, they note that health care presents
unusually complex conceptual issues for the analysis of elasticity of demand.
Presumably adequate care for a variety of health conditions can be secured
inside or outside a hospital and can include different degrees of convenience
and amenities, and outpatient care can be secured from health specialists or
generalists; the costs of these various forms of care tend to differ significantly. Consequently, a reduction in expenditures for care can reflect different sources and types of care purchased without requiring the conclusion
that the care received is inadequate. Put simply, given the current level of
knowledge about the relationship between health care and health outcomes,
one cannot assume a priori that the purchase of more expensive care is better
and that the purchase of less expensive care is worse (Enthoven, 1980; Feldstein, 1979).

With these caveats about the difficulty in measuring elasticity in demand
for health care in mind, some data from the RHS study are useful for investigating economic factors affecting variations in demand for health care
among persons aged 58 to 67 in the period from 1968 to 1972. Consider, for
example, Table 8.6. The older consumer in the sample who is presumably in
the best situation to make rational decisions about investing in health care is
an educated male who was not functionally impaired and not economically
impaired at all three observations ($N = 227$). From 1968 to 1972, for those
reporting health expenditures of one dollar or more, mean medical bills
decreased slightly. In an analysis not shown, the health share of these subjects
increased 75 percent, but this relatively large percentage increase nonetheless
produced a health share of 3.5 percent, which remained well below the study
population average. In contrast is the individual in the worst position to make
rational decisions about investing in health — the uneducated female who was
significantly impaired functionally (IFI about 2.25) and economically
impaired at all three observations ($N = 383$). These persons decreased their
real dollar investment by 17 percent, and the health share decreased 25 percent (from 15.4 percent to 11.5 percent). Income affected demand for care in

TABLE 8.6. Experience of Most Advantaged and Least Advantaged RHS Consumers, 1968 and 1972

1968	Medical Bills	Personal Expenditures	Expenses/ Bills [a] Ratio	Days Hospitalized	Doctor Visits
Median					
All reporting	$ 85	$ 71		0.00	11.0
Reporting $1 or more	104	94			
Most advantaged					
Mean					
All reporting	$251	$135		0.09	8.5
Reporting $1 or more	287	155	.854		
Median					
All reporting	$ 57	$ 5		0.00	13.0
Reporting $1 or more	97	28			
Least advantaged					
Mean					
All reporting	$199	$116		0.15	13.5
Reporting $1 or more	280	150	.77		
1972					
Median					
All reporting	$113	$ 91		0.00	2.0
Reporting $1 or more	128	98			
Most advantaged					
Mean					
All reporting	$259	$181		0.11	3.6
Reporting $1 or more	284	198	.84		
Median					
All reporting	$ 45	$ 25		0.00	4.0
Reporting $1 or more	94	46			
Least advantaged					
Mean					
All reporting	$140	$108		0.18	7.3
Reporting $1 or more	203	146	.80		

Source: Retirement History Study, 1969–73 interviews.

[a] This is the mean of the ratio of expenditures to bills for individuals. It is not the ratio of mean expenditures to mean medical bills.

both instances. The most economically secure individuals made investments in the maintenance of health at a level slightly below that required to keep up with increased cost of care. The economically impaired decreased their purchase of health care significantly. As we will show later, these decreases in relative investments in health care are not artifacts of increased insurance coverage.

Similarly, individuals who were in the work force at all three observations and whose constant dollar income remained stable decreased their investment in health care by 4.5 percent and their health share by 2.6 percent. For those out of the work force at all three observations, investment in health care in constant dollars decreased by 23 percent and the health share decreased by 9.6 percent. In both instances there is evidence that variation in demand can be explained at least in part by income changes.

Additional evidence of the effects of income on demand for health care is provided by an analysis of the behavior of individuals experiencing an illness resulting in hospitalization. A subgroup ($N = 490$) of economically unimpaired individuals in 1969 experienced hospitalization prior to their report of expenditures for health care in 1971. For these individuals, personal expenditures in constant dollars increased by 85 percent and the health share increased by 122 percent. In contrast, a subgroup of economically impaired persons ($N = 240$) increased their investment in health care by 65 percent and their health share by 56 percent in response to an illness requiring hospitalization. An analogous pattern of differential increase in investment was found for the same subgroups in the period 1971–73, again illustrating the effect of income on elasticity in demand for care.

The availability of insurance is known to affect the purchase of health care. Insured persons purchased more health care than uninsured persons, as reflected both in total health expenditures and in out-of-pocket expenditures (Tables 8.4, 8.5). However, it should be noted that these expenditures tended to remain stable or to decrease between 1969 and 1972, a period in which increasing numbers of the study population became eligible for medicare and the medicaid program became operational, and a period in which the CPI of health care services was increasing rapidly. We note the relatively high proportion of out-of-pocket expenditures found in our analysis. We do not believe this proportion is an artifact of our measurement procedures, which involved determining the average ratio of out-of-pocket to total health expenditures of all subjects who had incurred any health expenses.

EFFECTS OF DIFFERENTIAL INVESTMENT IN HEALTH CARE

The inverse relationship between an average observed increase in functional incapacity with age and personal investment in health care invites exploration of the consequences of this relationship for the well-being of older adults. Further, individuals in the study of the same level of functional capacity varied considerably in their levels of health investments. Intuitively, investment in health care would be expected to increase the probability of improving functional status or at least moderating decline; failure to invest should predict an accelerated decline in functioning. The data in Table 8.7 appear to contradict these expectations.

Subjects were divided into three subgroups: (1) those whose total expenditures on health care were less than the 25th percentile, (2) those whose total expenditures on health care were between the 25th and 75th percentiles, and

TABLE 8.7. Total Health Care Bills and Change in Functional Status of RHS Respondents Between 1969 and 1971

Level of Expenditure	Index of Functional Impairment, 1969	Changes in Index of Functional Impairment Index, 1971		
		% Improved	% Same	% Worse
(1) Less than the 25th percentile	0	—	73.22	26.78
for level of expenditures,	1	43.71	37.53	18.77
by impairment status	2	50.35	29.08	20.57
	3	43.96	50.24	5.80
(2) Between the 25th and 75th	0	—	74.56	25.44
percentiles for level of	1	45.82	29.94	24.24
expenditures, by impairment	2	43.85	34.63	21.52
status	3	45.67	47.31	7.03
(3) More than the 75th percentile	0	—	59.51	40.49
for level of expenditures,	1	35.04	28.07	36.88
by impairment status	2	33.45	41.22	25.34
	3	36.84	58.85	4.31

Source: Retirement History Study, 1969–73 interviews.
Note: Does not include insurance premiums.

(3) those whose total expenditures on health care were more than the 75th percentile of the constant dollars spent on health care by persons in their functional status category (0 to 3). Within each subgroup, individuals were classified by functional status in 1969, and then the probability of maintaining or changing functional status in 1971 was determined. Review of Table 8.7 indicates a similar pattern of association between levels of investment and outcomes for each level of initial functional status at each level of investment. Those who invest most in health in 1969 do not consistently increase the probability of maintaining or improving functional status in 1971. The persistently high correlation between personal and total health expenditures would lead us to expect a similar conclusion if out-of-pocket expenditures were substituted for total expenditures in Table 8.7 and in an analysis not shown, this was the case. Further, in an analysis not shown, we decomposed the summary index of functional impairment into its component parts (physical health, subjective well-being, self-care capacity) and found no change in the relationships reported.

As further confirmation of the inability to modify decline in or improvement of functional status through level of investment in health care, a discriminant analysis (not shown) was performed to identify the factors related to functional status (four categorical outcomes, 0 to 3 on the index of functional impairment). Possible discriminants introduced included sociodemographic factors (e.g., gender and age), economic factors (e.g., constant dollar investments and health share), and previous status on the IFI. Of particular interest was the presence or absence of an economic variable as a discriminant. The principal discriminant of functional status in 1971 proved to be functional status index in 1969 (partial $R^2 = 0.36$) with total cash income in 1971 as a distant second (partial $R^2 = 0.03$). No other factor contributed significantly as a discriminant. A similar conclusion was reached in identifying the discriminants of functional status in 1973. Again the IFI in 1971 was the principal discriminant (partial $R^2 = 0.32$) of functional status in 1973, with no other factor accounting for more than 2 percent of the variance.

A regression analysis confirmed the conclusion of the discriminant analysis. With functional status controlled on the original scales (0–6) for each component of the index of functional impairment, health expenditures have a slight but substantively insignificant effect on functional status at a subsequent observation. A final observation about the relationship between differential investment and health care and functional capacity is provided by an analysis of factors related to the death of subjects in the study. Between 1969 and 1971 there were 245 males who died; another 277 died between 1971 and 1973. The IFI of these males who would die in the subsequent two years in both 1969 and 1971 was 1.48 (almost twice the index of the entire sample). It is worth noting that almost half of these persons in both subsamples (49 percent in 1969 and 46 percent in 1971) were in the low range of impairment (0 or 1). The investment in health care for both subsamples was, on average, high. In 1969, for example, personal expenditures for health care in constant dollars was \$328, some 141 percent of the study sample average, and the health share was 0.081 compared with the average sample share of 0.06. Similarly, in 1971, personal expenditures for those who would be dead by 1973 were \$265, some 126 percent of the sample average, and the health share was 0.094, compared with the average sample share of 0.07. These observations are additional reminders that relatively higher health care investments do not ensure survival, even among those who are relatively unimpaired functionally. The data also suggests that the high cost of health care in later life may be attributable substantially to the years immediately preceding death, not to the later years of life generally (see Roos and Shapiro, 1981; Vandenbos et al., 1982; Miners, 1981). For example, in 1976 the 6.4 percent of medicare enrollees who died in that year accounted for 31 percent of medicare payments. More recent estimates of the proportion of medicare costs attributable to the terminal year of life are much higher.

IMPLICATIONS FOR PUBLIC HEALTH POLICY

These data fill an important gap in the literature on the relationships among and expected changes over time in functional status, personal health care expenditures, elasticity in demand for care, and the consequences of differential health care investments for functional status among older adults.

Declines in functioning with age occur as expected, but these data provide two additional important observations. The trajectory of decline can be estimated not only for the total study population but also for various subgroups within this population (Table 8.1). Comparison of these trajectories emphasizes variability among subgroups of older adults both in the level of functioning at the initial observation in 1969 and in the average rate of decline over the subsequent four years. Males, for example, initially have a higher average level of functioning but also display a higher rate of decline. Economically unimpaired persons at the initial observation have an index of functional impairment which is one-third that of economically impaired persons but have a higher rate of decline; yet four years later the economically unimpaired have an IFI score which is only 40 percent that of the economically impaired. The importance of differentiation is reinforced further by the observation that average expectable decline in functioning masks important variations in functional status (Table 8.7). Decline is not unilinear for all individuals; some maintain or improve their functional status.

Evidence of differentiation among older individuals in initial functional status and in trajectories of decline is matched by evidence of differential personal investment in health care (Tables 8.2–8.6). On average, the share of cash income devoted to health care tends to increase slightly with age, but the observed average decreased constant dollar investment in health care is counterintuitive in the face of increasing functional impairment. There are competing possible explanations of these observations. One might argue that the decreased personal investment in health care is misleading; insurance or public funds might be available to the individual so that total health care expenditures for individuals might compensate for declining personal investment. The evidence presented in Tables 8.4, 8.5, and 8.6 appears to contradict this explanation. Alternatively, one might argue, following Menefee (1980), that the observed decline in personal investment in health is predicted by a human capital perspective. This perspective, Menefee argues, suggests that older adults are increasingly aware that the cost of attempting to slow or reverse expectable decline in functioning through investment in health care has progressively lower utility. Such an assessment might be reinforced by realistic expectations derived from experience about the probability of declining function with age, experience with the limited ability of expensive, high-technology health care to reverse or slow functional decline, or both.

These data do not provide a definite test of these alternative explanations but the data are suggestive. There is evidence of elasticity of demand for care related to income. Older persons with the greater economic resources make greater investments in health care over time. Regardless of available personal economic resources, however, investment of actual total constant dollars in health care declines with age and over time in the RHS study population. Further, the evidence indicates that the level of investment in health care does not have a demonstrable effect, on average, on stabilizing or reversing functional decline. Health economists have noted increasing evidence of what has been called "flat of the curve" investment in high-technology health care; that is, there is evidence of decreased marginal utility of investments in health care in producing health (Enthoven, 1980; Feldstein, 1979).

Evidence from the RHS data does not provide a clear picture of the calculations used by older adults as they assess the utility of investing personal resources in health care. These data do invite the inference that the utility of investing in health care personally is perceived to decrease with age. However, factors other than personal investment in health care clearly are required to explain how observed differential maintenance, improvement, or decline of functioning occurs. The discriminant analysis reported above, which indicates that prior functioning is the best predictor of subsequent functioning, invites an additional inference. The differential risk of illness and impairment in the later years probably reflects genetic factors, life-style and behavioral factors known to be related to health, and the quality and quantity of health care received. These factors interact over the life course and account for the observed differences in levels of functioning and the trajectories of decline observed in the later years. These differences and trajectories of functional decline may be influenced relatively little — as they appear to be — by differential levels of personal investment in health care observed among older persons.

The implications of these data for public policy warrant careful consideration. The evidence is not an argument for reducing personal and public investments in health care for older adults. Appropriate health care can demonstrably reduce pain and suffering in acute and chronic illness. Whether health care — or more specifically the kind of health care currently available for purchase — has a reasonable probability of stabilizing or improving functional capacity is another matter. The evidence presented here suggests that it does not and that it is perhaps so perceived by older adults and possibly also by health care providers as they decide to invest their personal resources in health care. This is the case not only for older persons in general but also for those presumably in a position to make the most rational decisions regarding their investments in health care — educated persons with the resources to make such investments if they choose to do so. Further, we have called attention to the very high cost of health care in the terminal years of life in contrast to average health cost of older populations. A very high proportion of medicare expenditures, for example, is made on behalf of older individuals hospitalized in the final years of life.

Inflation in the cost of health care affects the quantity of care demanded, and this effect is accentuated by differences in income. Older persons with limited economic resources decrease their personal investment in health care over time more than those with greater economic resources. But even when health insurance and personal financial resources are available, the evidence indicates that older adults tend to reduce their investment in health care over time. Inflation in the cost of health care and low income affect the demand for health care, but the reduction in personal investment in health noted in our analysis appears to reflect more than simply personal income and the cost of care. Observed differences in levels of personal investment in health among the older adults studied do not have a demonstrable beneficial effect on functioning; reduced investment in health care may well reflect awareness on the part of older adults that this is so. In the future attention should focus less on how much is spent by older adults on health and more on what types of health care are purchased and the effects of the types of care chosen on stabilizing or improving functioning in the later years. Finally, attention should focus on differentiating personal investment in health care generally and public investment in health care for the terminally ill.

The tendency of the aging Retirement History Study panelists to decrease expenditures for health (both out-of-pocket and totally) in spite of increasing functional impairment was observed at a time when federal policy was designed to increase access to care by older persons through insurance (medicare) and public provision of care (medicaid). At the beginning of the 1980s, cost containment clearly had become an objective of federal health care policy. This concern is reflected in changes in medicare regulations requiring greater participation by elderly consumers in sharing the cost of care and restrictions of services covered. States have been required to increase their share of medicaid payments.

Although the effects of these changes on patterns of health care utilization and on the health of older adults remain to be determined, the evidence from the Retirement History Study reviewed here provides a baseline for comparison. Although the availability of health insurance or public payment for services is known to increase utilization of health care, one would reasonably anticipate from data presented here that in the 1980s the utilization of care by older individuals would, on average, decrease and that the out-of-pocket cost of care utilized would increase. Based on the analysis of data reviewed in this chapter, we are not at all confident that decreased functional status will follow. If decreased functional status is the outcome, it is most likely to occur not for older adults generally but for those older adults who are economically disadvantaged and hence have limited capacity to pay increased out-of-pocket costs for health care.

9 Summary of Inflation Effects and the Outlook for the 1980s

Real income of the elderly rose during the inflationary decade of the 1970s, and their relative income improved compared to other age groups. This gain in well-being during a period of rapidly rising prices contradicts the belief that older persons were especially vulnerable to the loss of real income with inflation. Current inflation protection of the elderly stems from continued earnings that rise to reflect price increases, government transfers that are explicitly or implicitly indexed to price increases, the decision by firms to award increases in postretirement benefits, and rising nominal returns to financial and real assets.

Careful analysis of the experience of the 1970s will enable us to examine potential inflation effects during the 1980s. The recent past may provide a guide for the future if the income trends can be explained and general relationships identified. The findings and discussion of earlier chapters, and the changing economic and political environment, provide the basis for an assessment of the effects inflation may have on the economic well-being of the elderly in the future.

INFLATION AND THE WELL-BEING OF THE ELDERLY: A REVIEW OF RESEARCH FINDINGS

The hypothesis that the elderly have been adversely affected by inflation relative to the population at large in the past decade is rejected by the evidence. The use of several data sets and price indexes shows that the real income of older persons has not fallen during recent periods of high inflation. The Retirement History Study and the Panel Study of Income Dynamics showed that income declined with age, as expected; the level of income fell at retirement, and earnings declined in importance, while pensions and social security comprised an increasing share of family income. An important finding is that real income appeared to be constant in the years prior to retirement and in the retirement period. Other studies and aggregate data revealed a favorable trend in the well-being of persons 65 and over; the real and relative income of persons 65 and older improved during the past two decades and the incidence of poverty among the elderly dropped sharply.

120

The popular notion that the elderly are harmed by inflation is in error principally because the basic premise that older persons live on fixed incomes is incorrect. Chapters 5 and 6 indicate that most of the sources of income of the elderly rose in nominal value when prices increased. Social security and many other governmental cash benefits have been automatically indexed to the increase in the consumer price index. Market wages and returns to assets were also responsive to price fluctuations. The analysis in these chapters shows that nominal income of the elderly was not fixed but rose when prices increased. The evidence suggests that the nominal income of older persons rose more rapidly than prices. But the elderly are not a homogeneous group, and various groups differ in their levels and sources of income. The low-income elderly have had the most protection from inflation because of the indexation of government transfers. Higher-income persons with income from private pensions have probably been the most vulnerable to loss in real income.

One problem with assessing trends in real income is in determining the appropriate index to deflate nominal income. Chapters 1 and 2 illustrate the conceptual issues involved in this procedure, and Chapter 3 discusses a series of potential deflators. For most purposes, the consumer price index is used to adjust transfer benefits even though it theoretically overstates the amount of adjustment required to maintain the same level of living. Revised indexes employing rent equivalencies instead of the current CPI treatment of housing indicate that the CPI overstates the rise in prices for all consumers, including the elderly. A review of recent literature finds only minor differences in the CPI and specially constructed indexes for the elderly. In addition, substantial variation is noted in price increases among various subgroups of the elderly. Thus, the consumer price index is a reasonable measure to deflate nominal income in determining trends in real income of the elderly without overstating the increase in real income.

Chapters 7 and 8 examine data from the Consumer Expenditure Survey and the Retirement History Study to determine changes in consumption and expenditure patterns. Analysis of the CES indicated increases in consumption for most subgroups for the elderly between 1972 and 1973. Both sets of data reflect life-cycle patterns of declining income and expenditures when cohorts were followed over time. After controlling for age effects, the Retirement History Study data indicated an increase in the level of real expenditures for selected food, housing, and medical items between 1970 and 1972. Small decreases were observed between 1968 and 1970 and again between 1972 and 1974.

Chapters 1 and 2 indicate that a comprehensive concept of well-being should measure the ability of persons to purchase and consume goods, services, and leisure time. Danziger et al. (1982) show the importance of a series of such adjustments to income in the determination of the relative income of the elderly in 1973. They find that the mean income of the elderly rises from 48.6 percent of the cash income of the nonelderly to 90 percent when they adjusted for consumption of the flow of service from durable goods, direct taxes, family size and composition, and the age of each household member. Their adjustments do not include the value of in-kind benefits or the value of the greater amount of leisure time enjoyed by the elderly.

The improving well-being of the elderly, the trend in family cash income, changes in work patterns, and rising in-kind government benefits are briefly reviewed below. Tying these components together provides a detailed picture of the trend in the well-being of older persons.

The median real cash income of families whose head is aged 65 or older rose by almost 100 percent between 1950 and 1980. Compared to families with heads aged 45 to 54, the relative income of elderly families fell by 13.4 percent during the 1950s and by 6.7 percent in the 1960s before rising by 13.4 percent during the 1970s (see Table 4.12). During these decades, the CPI rose by 23.3 percent, 31.1 percent, and 112.4 percent, respectively. Thus, the loss in relative income was greatest when inflation was the lowest and there was a significant gain in relative income during the high inflation decade of the 1970s. The rise in relative income of the elderly may have occurred because of the virtual cessation of real economic growth during the 1970s, which stopped the growth in the real income of workers. By contrast, the real income of the elderly continued to rise with increases in the real value of government transfers.

Households can vary the way they allocate their time in order to influence their levels of living. For example, time can be used to produce goods consumed by the family. These goods may be in the form of meal preparation, home repairs, leisure time, and so forth. Thus, time at home is valued by individuals and is an important aspect of family well-being. The trends in cash income presented above do not include changes in time at home that affect family welfare.

Age-specific labor force participation rates are one measure of the intensity of market work by a population group and hence are an indirect measure of time available for home activities. Table 9.1 shows that the labor force participation rate for males aged 65 and over fell by 60 percent between 1950 and 1981. Participation rates for older women also declined slightly during this period. Thus, the rise in real income discussed earlier understates the increase in welfare due to significant increases in home time by the elderly. By contrast, the total work effort of persons aged 45 to 54 increased during these three decades, with all the increase in work effort attributable to increased participation of females. Therefore gains in income for this group overstate the rise in their well-being.

The cash income concept also ignores the value of in-kind transfers received by older persons. The federal government provides in-kind benefits

TABLE 9.1. Labor Force Participation Rates, 1950–81

Year	65 and Over		45–54	
	Males	Females	Males	Females
1950	45.8	9.7	95.8	37.9
1955	39.6	10.6	96.5	43.8
1960	33.1	10.8	95.7	49.8
1965	27.9	10.0	95.6	50.9
1970	26.8	9.7	94.3	54.4
1975	21.6	8.2	92.1	54.6
1979	19.9	8.3	91.4	58.3
1980	19.0	8.1	91.2	59.9
1981	18.4	8.0	91.4	61.1

Source: U.S. Department of Labor, *Employment and Training Report of the President, 1982* (Washington, D.C.: Government Printing Office, 1983), Table A-5, p. 157. Also ibid., *1980,* Table A-4, pp. 224–25.

TABLE 9.2. Real In-kind Transfers per Person Aged 65 and Older, 1970–81

Year	Medicare[a,b]		Federal Medicaid[c]
	Health Insurance	Supplemental Health Insurance	
1970	215.07	47.26	61.92
1975	278.70	69.72	76.72
1978	309.42	92.38	90.95
1981	370.54	126.54	83.90

[a] Values deflated by the medical component of the CPI (1967 = 100).
[b] Derived in Tables 5.6 and 5.7.
[c] Estimates for total medicaid expenditures for persons aged 65 and over are divided by population aged 65 and over. Expenditure estimates are from unpublished data from Califano (1978) and U.S. Congressional Budget Office, 1982. Nominal values are deflated by the medical component of the CPI.

in the form of health insurance and payment for medical services, food stamps and other nutritional programs, housing assistance, and energy assistance. Most of these programs have been initiated and expanded during the last two decades. For example, medicare and medicaid were established by legislation in 1965. Table 9.2 shows the significant increase in the real value of these benefits per older person during the 1970s. The combined real value of medicare and medicaid for the average older person rose from $324.25 in 1970 to $580.98 in 1981, an increase of 79 percent. Thus, inclusion of medical in-kind benefits with cash income would result in an even greater rise in the real income of the elderly during the 1970s. Other in-kind transfers have also increased in real value. The real value of the subsidy for food stamps rose from $95.16 per recipient in 1970 to $144.55 per recipient in 1981. Noncash compensation from employers has risen as a percentage of total compensation, so the effect of including in-kind income in the determination of the income of the elderly in relation to younger workers is unclear.

Thus, real cash income of the elderly has risen significantly during the past three decades. Adjusting cash income for increased leisure time and the growth of in-kind government transfers would indicate even greater gains for older persons. The growth in median real cash income of the elderly may also be understated because of a changing age composition of the older population. Since income is negatively related to age among older persons, an increasing proportion of the 65-and-over population that is over 75 or 85 would tend to slow the growth of the median income. The improvement in relative income is further understated because of the rising tax burden on younger workers, which has largely been avoided by the elderly.

One potential offset to these gains would be reductions in family in-kind or unreported cash transfers. We are unaware of any data that would enable one to calculate the size or direction of intrafamily resources over time. Another potential offset is the rate of change of prices faced by the elderly as compared to that of the general population. Existing studies and the research presented in this report indicate that the rates of changes in prices for the elderly are not substantially different from the general CPI, and recent evidence suggests that changes in the CPI may overstate the rise in prices faced by older consumers. Despite these potential offsets, the weight of the evidence clearly supports the argument that the real and relative well-being of the elderly were substantially improved during the 1970s, when inflation was at historically high rates.

UNCERTAINTY, INFLATION, AND WELL-BEING

In addition to changes in real income, there may be general effects of inflation on well-being that arise from its unpredictability and its distributional impact. Correctly anticipated inflation not entailing relative price changes causes people to hold less cash and make more frequent transactions, but these are relatively minor costs (Dornbusch and Fischer, 1981; Gordon, 1981). However, the rate of inflation is seldom fully anticipated, and higher rates of inflation tend to be accompanied by more relative price variability and by more variability in the rate of inflation (Vining and Elwertowski, 1976; Bordo, 1980; Parks, 1978; Cukierman, 1979; and Logue and Willet, 1976). When incorrectly anticipated, inflation is not built into the market transactions and institutions of an economy. This causes a basic loss in well-being and the sense of unfairness that makes inflation so unpopular.

The elderly share in the losses to the whole economy from not fully anticipating inflation. Two factors are involved in their relative loss. First, any group that tends to be more mistaken in its inflation expectations would lose more than other groups. Are the elderly more likely to be wrong in this regard than others? Given that they have had more experience with economic and political change and more time away from work to devote to market transactions, they may well do a better job of correctly anticipating inflation rates. Second, any group that has higher costs of adjusting its investment and consumption patterns to changes in relative prices implied by inflation would lose more. Are the elderly less flexible than others in adjusting income and consumption patterns? With more geographic mobility and more income from in-kind sources, including more time away from jobs to be used for leisure and consumption, the elderly may actually be more flexible in their buying and investment decisions. As a result, there is no presumption that the elderly suffer more of a loss in well-being than the general population faces with inflation.

INFLATION EFFECTS IN THE FUTURE

The analysis in this book has been devoted in large part to examining the historical record of improving real income of the elderly. This analysis will be useful for current policy-making only if general and continuing relationships can be shown to exist. These general responses can be used to discuss likely changes in the real income of the elderly through the remainder of the twentieth century. The objective of this section is to assess the findings of this research for their significance in projecting the future status of older persons.

Several age-specific patterns of consumption are revealed in Chapters 3, 7, and 8. These include the observation that older persons tend to spend a larger proportion of their income on food at home, medical care, and utilities. These budget shares have remained higher than similar shares for younger families. Reasons for these differences include lower income for older families, more time at home, and declining health with age. The perpetuation of different expenditure patterns by age creates the potential for greater rises in prices for goods consumed by one group.

There is no theoretical reason for the relative price changes of the 1970s to be repeated in the 1980s. For example, house prices rose rapidly during the 1970s but actually declined during the early 1980s. By contrast, food prices have risen more than the general CPI in some years and by less in others. The importance of relative price changes in determining changes in well-being should not be overlooked, but existing research of age-specific price indexes suggest that over reasonably long periods of time price increases for most demographic groups do not deviate substantially from the increase for the general population. Allowing for substitution in consumption would further moderate differences in relative price effects on the increase in the price of the market basket actually purchased.

These basic concepts and a review of recent price changes indicate that relative price changes within a general inflation will have only minor effects on the well-being of the elderly compared to that of other demographic groups. Thus, the primary issue governing the effect of inflation on real income of the elderly is the responsiveness of their incomes to rises in the general price level.

Earnings are determined by the amount of labor supplied and the market wage rate. Although labor supply is reduced with age, earnings remain an important source of income for many older persons. Real wages rise with growth in productivity. There is no theoretical reason that growth in the real wage rate for older workers would deviate from the general pattern of wage growth in the economy. This source of income should not cause changes in relative income between the elderly and the total population, and in general real wage growth will contribute to rising real income.

Real income from assets depends on changes in the rate of return to the items in an individual's investment portfolio compared to changes in the price level. Rates of return fluctuate over time, with price changes of houses, gold, diamonds, and stocks being recent examples. Speculation on future rates of return to assets held by the elderly is not an easy task and would require a complete macroeconomic forecasting model that predicted many price changes. The best hypothesis would seem to be that the elderly manage their portfolios in order to maximize the rate of return subject to risk and liquidity preferences. Their wealth allocation decisions will include expected future inflation rates and real rates of return to their assets. In such a framework, the expected effect of inflation on the real wealth of the elderly would not differ greatly from the effect on the rest of the population.

Continuing high rates of inflation may cause financial institutions to alter future payments to reflect price changes. For the elderly, one of the most important of these institutions is the employer pension system. Available evidence indicates that real pension benefits after retirement have declined with inflation, even though many firms provide ad hoc increases. A more formal adjustment mechanism might evolve if high rates of inflation continue for another decade.

Older persons also consume from their stock of durable goods, which includes the family car, home, furniture, appliances, and the like. The nominal value of consumption rises as the replacement costs of these durables rise. The real value of consumption from durable goods should be unaffected by general price increases. Thus, the relationships between these private sources of income and inflation indicate that nominal income rises with increases in consumer prices. This responsiveness of nominal income from private sources is due to general economic relationships and should continue in the future.

Income from governmental sources and its responsiveness to inflation depend on public policy decisions. These decisions are based on political considerations, relative income of the elderly, the tax burden on workers, and real economic growth. During the past three decades, there have been substantial increases in governmental transfers to the elderly. Social security retirement benefits and other governmental cash benefits as well as in-kind benefits have been increased rapidly in real value, and many of these programs are now explicitly indexed so that the nominal value of benefits rises automatically with increases in prices. Other benefits are increased by specific legislation. Since government transfers are now a major source of income for older persons, their responsiveness to price increases is an important determinant in the effect of inflation on their real income. In the post–World War II period, Congress has raised benefits sufficiently to offset potential losses due to inflation, and the use of indexation has reduced the legislative lag in benefit increases. These public policies have helped to produce rising real and relative income of older persons.

If these legislative patterns were to continue along with the existing indexation of programs, the trend in real income of the elderly established during the last two decades could be expected to continue. Many demographic, economic, and political factors are changing in ways that will limit the growth of transfer payments to the elderly. Social security legislation passed in 1983 represented the culmination of years of debate concerning the long-run and short-run financial crises the system was facing. This legislation provided for significant changes in the system and for a projected funding balance over the next seventy-five years. While the basic tenets of the program were left unchanged, the 1983 cost-of-living increase was delayed six months, and full indexing in the future was made conditional on the relative size of wage and price increases. These changes slightly reduce the inflation protection guaranteed through this major source of income to the elderly.

The aging of the population, especially in the first twenty years of the next century, will require a major restructuring of the total income maintenance system for the elderly. Either taxes must be raised substantially or benefits must be lowered or funds must be diverted from other national priorities. The 1983 social security legislation attempted to address this long-run problem by raising the age of eligibility for full benefits to 67 in the next century. In addition, medicare must be reevaluated to prevent rapidly rising costs from producing large deficits in the coming decades. Other transfers are likely to be affected by this demographic pressure, which may limit their future growth.

The increase in real benefits for older persons was stimulated in large measure by the belief that many older persons were destitute and that private methods would not provide the necessary transfers. The rise in real and relative income of the elderly along with a sharp decline in the incidence of poverty has reduced or eliminated some of the pressures for major new programs or increases in real benefits for the elderly in general. Recent budgetary initiatives have reduced benefits and tightened eligibility conditions for medicaid, food stamps, and other welfare programs that provide benefits to some older persons. Social security and medicare benefits also have been altered during the early 1980s. The cessation or slowing of the growth of real transfers to the elderly will reduce the likelihood that the experience of the 1970s, when the incomes of older persons rose significantly relative to the incomes of the general population, will be repeated in the future.

The trend toward indexation of these benefit programs is attributable to the commonly held view that the elderly live on fixed incomes. The full and perhaps over indexation of benefits during the past decade when real wages were falling has sharply changed this belief. As a result, indexation of social security, government pensions, and other transfers has been critically examined, and numerous proposals for their reductions have been made. Changes in the methods of indexing federal pensions and food stamps have already been enacted, and further modification of other indexing provisions seems likely during the 1980s. These changes will tend to lower future benefit increases in response to rising prices.

The changing political, economic, and demographic conditions in the early 1980s have produced modifications of government transfer programs that will limit their real growth and reduce the level of benefit increases in response to inflation. These changes in government policy will probably be sufficient to keep the relative income of the elderly from rising as it did in the 1970s. The growth in real income will also be moderated. Despite these recent changes in income maintenance programs, it should be noted that the poverty rate of persons aged 65 and over declined between 1980 and 1982, while the rate for the general population rose. In 1982, for the first time the poverty rate of the elderly was below the rate for the total population. In addition, the relative income of the elderly continued to rise. Thus, the improving relative well-being of the elderly that has been described during the 1970s has continued into the 1980s despite significant changes in public policy.

Thus we see that most sources of income of the elderly rise in response to increasing prices. There is no fundamental reason to expect real earnings or return to assets to fall with inflation. Nominal pension benefits have been increased, but in general these increases have lagged behind price changes; however, future institutional changes may moderate this effect. So income from private sources is not fixed in nominal terms, but instead tends to rise with increasing prices.

Most government transfer programs currently are indexed to reflect price increases automatically, but policy changes in the next few years may alter these provisions and reduce future benefits to older persons. Such changes in public policy would reduce the inflation protection of the elderly, as well as gains in their real income, in the short run. Over a longer period, the effects on incomes of the elderly will depend on private responses to government changes. Will children increase support for their aged parents? Will individuals alter life-cycle savings plans to provide increased wealth for their old age? Will the trend toward early retirement be reversed? Answers to these questions will determine the future levels of income of the elderly and the responsiveness of their income during inflationary periods.

References

Andersen, R., J. Kravits, and O. Anderson. 1975. *Equality in Health Services: Empirical Analysis in Social Policy.* Cambridge, Mass.: Ballinger.

Bankers Trust Company, Employee Benefits Division. 1980. *Corporate Pension Plan Study: A Guide for the 1980s.* New York: Bankers Trust Co.

Barnes, Roberta, and Shelia Zedlewski. 1981. "The Impact of Inflation on the Income and Expenditures of Elderly Families." Working Paper No. 1401-1. Washington, D.C.: Urban Institute, April.

Blinder, A. S. 1980. "The Consumer Price Index and the Measurement of Recent Inflation." *Brookings Papers on Economic Activity* 2:539–65.

Bordo, Michael David. 1980. "The Effects of Monetary Change on Relative Commodity Prices and the Role of Long-term Contracts." *Journal of Political Economy* 88 (December): 1088–109.

Borzilleri, Thomas. 1978. "The Need for a Separate Consumer Index for Older Persons." *Gerontologist* 18 (June): 230–36.

Borzilleri, Thomas. 1980. "In-kind Benefit Programs and Retirement." Paper prepared for the President's Commission on Pension Policy.

Boskin, Michael, and Michael Hurd. 1982. "Are Inflation Rates Different for the Elderly?" Working Paper No. 943. Cambridge, Mass.: National Bureau of Economic Research.

Braithwait, S. D. 1980. "The Substitution Bias of the Laspeyres Price Index: An Analysis Using Estimated Cost-of-living Indexes." *American Economic Review* 70 (March): 64–77.

Bridges, Benjamin, and Michael Packard. 1981. "Price and Income Changes for the Elderly." *Social Security Bulletin* 44 (January): 3–15.

Bunn, Julie A., and Jack E. Triplett. 1983. "Reconciling the CPI-U and the PCE Deflator: 3rd Quarter." *Monthly Labor Review* 106 (February): 37–38.

Cagan, P., and G. H. Moore. 1981. *The Consumer Price Index — Issues and Alternatives.* Washington, D.C.: American Enterprise Institute.

Califano, Joseph. 1978. "The Aging of America: Questions for the Four-generation Society." *Annuals of the American Academy of Political and Social Science* 438 (July): 96–107.

Campbell, Colin. 1976. *Over-indexed Benefits: The Decoupling Proposals for Social Security.* Washington, D.C.: American Enterprise Institute.

Cantrell, Rayford Stephen. 1982. "Urbanization, Mortality, and Income: An Economic Analysis of U.S. Urban-Rural Mortality." Ph.D. dissertation, North Carolina State University.

Clark, Robert. 1977. *The Role of Private Pensions in Maintaining Living Standards in Retirement.* Washington, D.C.: National Planning Association.

Clark, Robert, Steven Allen, and Daniel Sumner. 1983. "Inflation and Pension Benefits." U.S. Department of Labor, Contract No. J-9-P-1-0074, August.

Clark, Robert, and David Barker. 1981. *Reversing the Trend Toward Early Retirement.* Washington, D.C.: American Enterprise Institute.

Clark, Robert, Stephan Gohmann, and Daniel Sumner. 1981. "Wages and Hours of Work of Elderly Men." Faculty Working Paper No. 4, North Carolina State University, December.

Clark, Robert, and Thomas Johnson. 1980. "Retirement in the Dual Career Family." Final Report for Social Security Administration Grant No. 10-P-90543-4-02, June.

Clark, Robert, and Ann McDermed. 1982. "Inflation, Pension Benefits, and Retirement." *Journal of Risk and Insurance* 49 (March): 19–38.

Clark, Robert, and John Menefee. 1981. "Federal Expenditures for the Elderly." *Gerontologist* 21 (April): 132–37.

Cook, Thomas. 1981. *Public Retirement Systems, Summaries of Public Retirement Plans Covering Colleges and Universities.* New York: TIAA-CREF.

Cukierman, Alex. 1979. "The Relationship Between Relative Prices and the General Price Level: A Suggested Interpretation." *American Economic Review,* 69 (June): 444–47.

Danziger, Sheldon, Jacques van der Gaag, Eugene Smolensky, and Michael Taussig. 1982. "Implications of the Relative Economic Status of the Elderly for Transfer Policy." Paper prepared for Brookings Institution Conference on Retirement and Aging, Washington, D.C., October.

Deaton, Angus, and John Muellbauer. 1980. *Economics and Consumer Behavior.* Cambridge: Cambridge University Press.

Dornbusch, Rudiger, and Stanley Fischer. 1981. *Macroeconomics.* New York: McGraw-Hill.

Duke University Center for the Study of Aging and Human Development. 1978. *The OARS Methodology. 2d ed.* Durham, N.C.: Duke University.

Enthoven, A. C., 1980. *Health Plan.* Reading, Mass.: Addison-Wesley.

"Family Budgets." 1968–81. *Monthly Labor Review,* various issues.

Feder, Judith, John Holahan, and Theodore Marmar. 1980. *National Health Insurance: Conflicting Goals and Policy Choices.* Washington, D.C.: Urban Institute.

Feldstein, M. J. 1979. *Health Care Economics.* New York: Wiley.

Ferber, R. 1966. *The Reliability of Consumer Reports of Financial Assets and Debts.* Urbana: University of Illinois Press.

Fillenbaum, Gerda, and L. Landerman. 1981. *Application of a Functional Classification System.* Final report to the Social Security Administration. Durham, N.C.: Duke University Center for the Study of Aging and Human Development.

Fillenbaum, Gerda, and George Maddox. 1977. *Assessing the Functional Status of LRHS Participants.* Technical Report No. 2. Durham, N.C.: Duke University Center for the Study of Aging and Human Development, September.

Fletcher, Stanley McCaul. 1981. "Economic Implications of Changing Household Food Expenditure Patterns." Ph.D. dissertation, North Carolina State University.

Fox, Alan. 1979. "Earnings Replacement of Retired Couples." *Social Security Bulletin* 42 (January): 17–39.

Fries, J. 1981. "Aging, Natural Death, and the Compression of Morbidity." In A. Somers and D. Fabian (eds.), *The Geriatric Imperative.* New York: Appleton-Century-Crofts.

Gallo, Anthony, Larry E. Salathe, and William T. Boehm. 1979. *Senior Citizens: Food Expenditure Patterns and Assistance.* Agricultural Economic Report, no. 426. Washington, D.C.: U.S. Department of Agriculture. June.

Gillingham, Robert, and Walter Lane. 1982. "Changing the Treatment of Shelter Costs for Homeowners in the CPI." *Monthly Labor Review* 105 (June): 9–14.

Gordon, Robert. 1981. *Macroeconomics.* Boston: Little, Brown, & Co.

Greenough, William, and Francis King. 1976. *Pension Plans and Public Policy.* New York: Columbia University Press.

Grimaldi, Paul. 1982. "Measured Inflation and the Elderly, 1973–81." *Gerontologist* 22 (August): 347–53.

Grossman, M. 1972. *The Demand for Health.* New York: Columbia University Press.

Gustman, Alan L., and Thomas L. Steinmeier. 1981. "Partial Retirement and the Analysis of Retirement Behavior." Working Paper No. 763. Cambridge, Mass.: National Bureau of Economic Research.

Hamermesh, Daniel S. 1982a. "Consumption During Retirement: The Missing Link in the Lifecycle." Working Paper No. 930. Cambridge, Mass.: National Bureau of Economic Research.

———. 1982b. "Lifecycle Effects on Consumption and Retirement." Working Paper No. 976. Cambridge, Mass.: National Bureau of Economic Research.

Haug, M. 1981. "Age and Medical Care Utilization Patterns." *Journal of Gerontology* 36: 103–11.

Hay Associates. 1981. "Hay-Huggins Noncash Compensation Comparison." Philadelphia: Hay Associates.

Henderson, James, and Richard Quandt. 1980. *Microeconomic Theory.* New York: McGraw-Hill.

Hewitt Associates. 1981. "Post-retirement Pension Increases Among Major U.S. Employers." New York: Hewitt Associates.

Hickey, T. 1980. *Health and Aging.* Monterey, Calif.: Brooks/Cole.

Hiemstra, Steve. 1981. Personal communication with Ronald Schrimper.

Holtzmann, A. G., and E. O. Olsen. 1978. *The Economics of Private Demand for Outpatient Health Care.* Washington, D.C.: U.S. Department of Health, Education, and Welfare.

Hurd, Michael, and John Shoven. 1982a. "The Economic Status of the Elderly." Working Paper No. 914. Cambridge, Mass.: National Bureau of Economic Research.

———. 1982b. "Real Income and Wealth of the Elderly." *American Economic Review* 72 (May): 314–18.

Irelan, Lola. 1972. "Retirement History Study: Introduction." *Social Security Bulletin* 35 (November): 3–8.

Kaplan, Robert. 1977. *Indexing Social Security.* Washington, D.C.: American Enterprise Institute.

King, Francis. 1982. "Indexing Retirement Benefits." *Gerontologist* 22 (December): 488–92.

Layard, P. R. G., and A. A. Walters. 1978. *Microeconomic Theory.* New York: McGraw-Hill.

Logue, Dennis, and Thomas Willet. 1976. "A Note on the Relation Between the Rate and Variability of Inflation." *Economica* 43 (May): 151–58.

Maddox, G. L. 1981. "Measuring the Well-being of Older Adults." In A. Somers and

D. Fabian (eds.), *The Geriatric Imperative,* pp. 117–36. New York: Appleton-Century-Crofts.

Maddox, G. L., G. Fillenbaum, and L. George. 1979. "Extending the Uses of LRHS Data Set." *Public Data Use* 7:57–61.

Mansfield, Edwin. 1979. *Microeconomics.* New York: Norton & Co.

Marquis, K. 1980. "Hospital Stay Response Error from the Health Insurance Study's Dayton Baseline Survey." RAND (R-2555-HEW). Santa Monica, Calif.: Rand Corporation.

Menefee, John. 1980. "The Demand for Health and Retirement." In R. L. Clark (ed.), *Retirement Policy in an Aging Society,* pp. 18–51. Durham, N.C.: Duke University Press.

Menefee, John, Bea Edwards, and Sylvester Schieber. 1981. "Analysis of Nonparticipation in the SSI Program." *Social Security Bulletin* 38 (June): 3–21.

Michael, R. 1979. "Variations Across Households in the Rate of Inflation." *Journal of Money, Credit, and Banking* 11 (February): 32–46.

Miller, Roger Leroy. 1982. *Intermediate Microeconomics.* New York: McGraw-Hill.

Miners, M. 1981. "Shifting the Burden." Paper presented at the annual meeting of the American Public Health Association.

Moon, Marilyn. 1977. *The Measuring of Economic Welfare: Its Application to the Aged Poor.* New York: Academic Press.

———. 1979. "The Incidence of Poverty Among the Elderly." *Journal of Human Resources* 14 (Spring): 211–21.

Moon, Marilyn, and Eugene Smolensky. 1977. *Improving Measures of Economic Well-being.* New York: Academic Press.

Motley, Dena K. 1975. "Paying for Health Care in the Years Before Retirement." *Social Security Bulletin* 38: 25–42.

Munnell, Alicia. 1977. *The Future of Social Security.* Washington, D.C.: Brookings Institution.

———. 1979. *Pensions for Public Employees.* Washington, D.C.: National Planning Association.

Murray, Janet H. 1978. "Changes in Food Expenditures, 1969–73: Findings from the Retirement History Study." *Social Security Bulletin* 41 (July).

Myers, Robert. 1975. *Social Security.* Homewood, Ill.: Irwin.

National Center for Health Services Research. 1977. *Controlling the Cost of Health Care.* NCHSR Policy Research Series, 77-3182. Washington, D.C.: U.S. Department of Health, Education, and Welfare.

Newhouse, J. P., and C. E. Phelps. 1973. "Price and Income Elasticities for Medical Care Services." In M. Perlman (ed.), *The Economics of Health and Medical Care,* pp. 139–61. New York: Wiley.

Okun, Arthur. 1970. "Inflation: The Problems and Prospects Before Us." In Arthur Okun, Henry Fowler, and Milton Gilbert (eds.), *Inflation: The Problems It Creates and Policies It Requires,* pp. 3–56. New York: New York University Press.

O'Neill, June. 1978. Unpublished data prepared for the Congressional Budget Office. Estimates summarized in James Story and Gary Hendricks, *Retirement Income Issues in an Aging Society.* Washington, D.C.: Urban Institute, December 1979.

Paglin, Morton. 1980. *Poverty and Transfers In-kind.* Stanford, Calif.: Hoover Institution Press.

Parks, Richard. 1978. "Inflation and Relative Price Variability." *Journal of Political Economy* 86 (February): 79–95.

Prochaska, Fred J., and R. A. Schrimper. 1973. "Opportunity Cost of Time and Other Socioeconomic Effects on Away-From-Home Food Consumption." *American Journal of Agricultural Economics* 55 (November): 595–603.

Reinecke, John A. 1971. "Expenditures of Two-person Units and Individuals After Age 55." Staff Paper No. 9. Washington, D.C.: U.S. Department of Health, Education, and Welfare, Social Security Administration, May.

Roos, N. P., and E. Shapiro. 1981. "The Manitoba Longitudinal Study of Aging: Preliminary Findings on Health Care Utilization." *Medical Care* 19: 664–57.

Rosen, Sherwin. 1981. "Some Arithmetic of Social Security." Paper presented at American Enterprise Institute Conference, Washington, D.C., June.

Schwenk, F. N. 1981. "Two Measures of Inflation: The Consumer Price Index and the Personal Consumption Expenditure Implicit Price Deflator." *Family Economics Review,* Winter, 13–18.

Shanas, E., and G. Maddox. 1976. "Aging, Health, and the Organization of Health Resources." In R. Binstock and E. Shanas (eds.), *Handbook of Aging and the Social Sciences,* pp. 592–618. New York: Van Nostrand Reinhold.

Smeeding, Timothy. 1982. *Alternative Methods of Valuing Selected In-kind Transfer Benefits and Measuring Their Impact on Poverty.* Technical Paper No. 50. Washington, D.C.: U.S. Bureau of the Census, April.

Stevens, Robert, and Rosemary Stevens. 1974. *Welfare Medicine in America.* New York: Free Press.

Strate, John. 1982. "Post-retirement Benefit Increases in State Pension Plans." Policy Center on Aging, Waltham, Mass.: Brandeis University.

Thompson, Gayle. 1978. "The Impact of Inflation on the Private Pension Benefits of Retirees, 1970–74: Findings from the Retirement History Study." *Social Security Bulletin* 41 (November): 16–25.

Tilove, Robert. 1976. *Public Employee Pension Funds.* New York: Columbia University Press.

Tomek, William. 1977. "Empirical Analysis of the Demand for Food: A Review." In Robert Raunikar (ed.), *Food Demand and Consumption Behavior.* Athens, Ga.: S-119 Southern Regional Research Committee, State Agricultural Experiment Stations and the Farm Foundation, March.

Torrey, Barbara. 1982. "Guns vs. Canes: The Fiscal Implications of an Aging Population." *American Economic Review* 72 (May): 309–13.

Triplett, J. E. 1981. "Reconciling the CPI and PCE Deflator." *Monthly Labor Review* 104 (September): 3–15.

U.S. Bureau of Labor Statistics. 1970. *Three Budgets for a Retired Couple in Urban Areas of the United States, 1967–68.* Bulletin No. 1570-6. Washington, D.C.: Government Printing Office, May.

U.S. Congressional Budget Office. 1977. *Poverty Status of Families Under the Alternative Definitions.* Background Paper No. 17 (revised). Washington, D.C.: Government Printing Office.

U.S. Congressional Budget Office. 1982. *Work and Retirement: Options for Continued Employment of Older Workers.* Washington, D.C.: Government Printing Office, July.

U.S. Congressional Research Service. 1981. *Indexation of Federal Programs.* Washington, D.C.: Government Printing Office.

U.S. Department of Commerce, Bureau of Economic Analysis. 1981. *The National Income and Product Amounts of the United States, 1929–76 Statistical Tables.* September.

U.S. Department of Commerce, Bureau of Economic Analysis. 1982. *Survey of Current Business* 62, no. 7 (July).

U.S. Department of Commerce, Bureau of Economic Analysis. 1983. *Survey of Current Business* 63, no. 7 (July).

U.S. Social Security Administration. 1980. *Social Security Bulletin: Annual Statistical Abstract, 1977–79.* Washington, D.C.: Government Printing Office.

Upp, Melinda. 1983. "Relative Importance of Various Income Sources of the Aged, 1980." *Social Security Bulletin* 46 (January): 3–10.

Vandenbos, G., P. De Leon, and M. Pollok. 1982. "An Alternative to Medical Care for the Terminally Ill." *American Psychologist* 37: 1245–48.

Vining, Daniel, and Thomas Elwertowski. 1976. "The Relationship Between Relative Prices and the General Price Level." *American Economic Review* 66 (September): 699–708.

Wan, Thomas T. H. 1982. *Stressful Life Events, Social Supports Networks, and Gerontological Health.* Lexington, Mass.: Lexington Books.

Watts, H. W. 1980. "Special Panel Suggests Changes in BLS Family Budget Program." *Monthly Labor Review* 103 (December): 3–10.

White House Conference on Aging. 1982. *1981 Final Report,* vol. 1. N. p.

Index

About the Authors

Robert L. Clark is a professor in the Department of Economics and Business at North Carolina State University and a senior fellow at the Center for the Study of Aging and Human Development at Duke University. Among his books are *Economics of Individual and Population Aging* (with Joseph Spengler) and *Sex, Age, and Work: The Changing Composition of the Labor Force* (with Juanita Kreps). **George L. Maddox** is director and senior fellow at the Center for the Study of Aging and Human Development at Duke University and professor of sociology and medical sociology at Duke University and Duke University Medical Center. He is author of *Perspectives on Aging: Exploding the Myth* and editor (with H. Thomae) of *New Perspectives on Old Age: A Message to Decision Makers.* **Ronald A. Schrimper** is professor of economics and business at North Carolina State University. **Daniel A. Sumner** is associate professor of economics at North Carolina State.